TRADITIONAL FOLK VETERINARY MEDICINES

TRADITIONAL FOLK VETERINARY MEDICINES

TRADITIONAL FOLK VETERINARY MEDICINES

S.S. Katewa
P.K. Galav
Anita Jain

Laboratory of Ethnobotany and Agrostology,
Department of Botany, University College of Science,
M.L. Sukhadia University
Udaipur (Raj.)

SCIENTIFIC
PUBLISHERS (INDIA)
www.scientificpub.com

Published by:
Scientific Publishers (India)
5-A, New Pali Road, P.O. Box 91,
Jodhpur – 342 001 (India)

E-mail: info@scientificpub.com
www.scientificpub.com

ISBN: 978-81-7233-665-3

Lasertype set : Rajesh Ojha
Printed in India

PREFACE

Livestock health is a major problem facing farmers and herders throughout India. Veterinarians are few in remote areas and the cost of modern treatment is expensive, inaccessible and sometimes inappropriate because it is not sustainable in the prevailing socioeconomic conditions. This situation has seen the rise and application of indigenous and traditional livestock treatment practices as the most immediate solution. This practice is commonly referred to as Ethnoveterinary and is the subject of this book.

Ethnoveterinary knowledge (sometimes also called veterinary anthropology) deals with folk beliefs, knowledge, skills, methods and practices pertaining to the health care of animals.

Ethnoveterinary knowledge is part of indigenous knowledge and as an integral part of traditional knowledge it forms part of a community cultural heritage.

Ethnoveterinary medicine can make an important contribution to improving the veterinary healthcare infrastructure in India and increase the productivity of Indian livestock.

There has been a spurt of publications on traditional medicinal plants related to human ailments but only few publications are available related to ailments of animals. Our team has a mission to work with dedication in the service of mute animals.

The present work on alternative medicine related to our age old heritage of traditional veterinary practices will eventually help millions of farmers for treating large number of common animal diseases and thoroughly contribute in livestock production and overall rural development. It is time now to supplement our validated traditional knowledge and present this great contribution to the nation, and train our veterinarians and herbalists / healers to preserve and harness nature in services of the rural masses and the mute animals, by developing cheap, tested, potent, easily and readily available herbal remedies to be in the service of animal health and production, by offering cheap, easily available, harmless plant medicines, of which many are validated and are highly adoptable.

The chief purpose of this book is to provide information about therapeutic uses of the herbs of forests and thus foster an interest in the so-called plant derived "Wonder Drugs". The information on the plant species includes the latest valid botanical name, with vernacular names in use in the area covered; a systematic and brief botanical description; phenology giving the months of flowering and fruiting and ethnoveterinary uses. This book is profusely illustrated to aid recognition of herbs described in this work. The present book is full of original ethnoveterinary observations taken during our ethnobotanical surveys. The book contains documentation of 265 ethnoveterinary plants which are used by the tribals and rural communities to treat various animal ailments. An attempt has been made to name the tribe making specific use and methods of preparation of the drug, dosage and duration have also been highlighted. Besides herbs, ethnoveterinary remedies based on animal and animal products and minerals are also given in the book.

People working in the field of Ayurveda, Pharmacology, Forestry, Conservation, Anthropology, Indian culture, History, Sociology, Ecology and Environmental biology would find this a very useful and informative book on folklore veterinary medicines. We may add that in spite of the care, which has been exercised in every way, there are bound to be some errors and omissions and we will appreciate having these brought to our notice by the users of this book. We and informants shall feel rewarded if any traditional herbal veterinary medicine documented in this book is developed into a modern drug of great therapeutic importance.

S.S. Katewa
P.K. Galav
Anita Jain

CONTENT

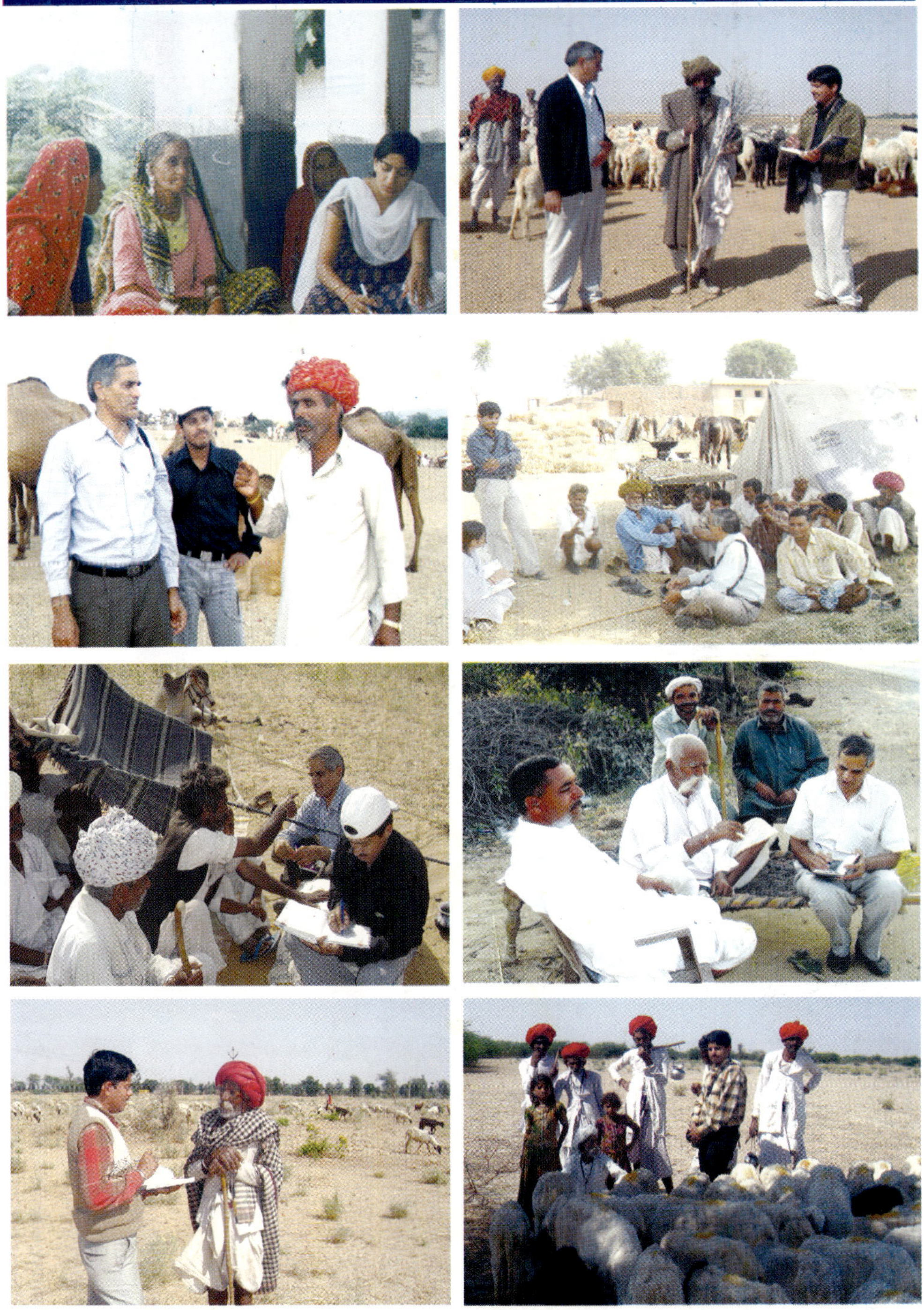

Authors interacting with indigenous healers (Raikas and Rebaris) of Rajasthan

Plate - 1

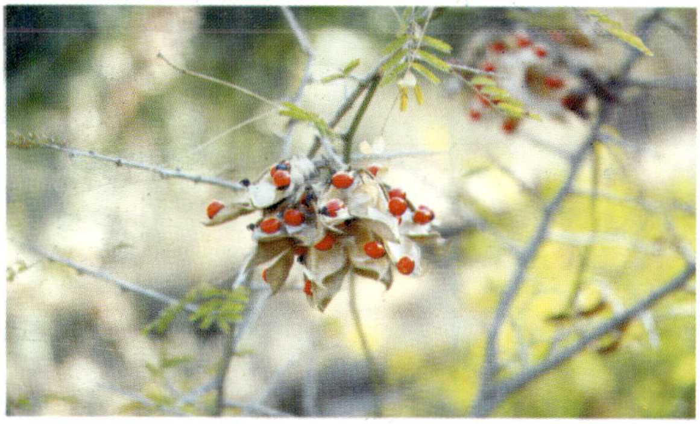

Abrus precatorius

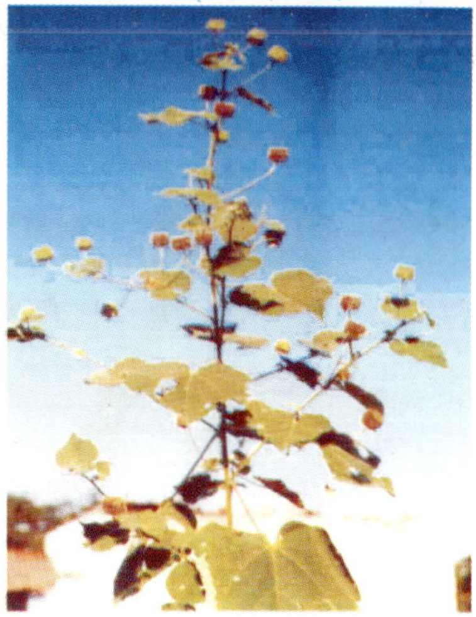

Abutilon indicum

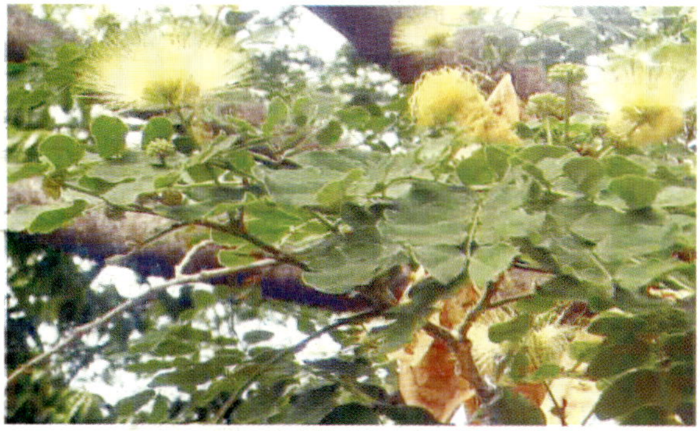

Albizia lebbeck

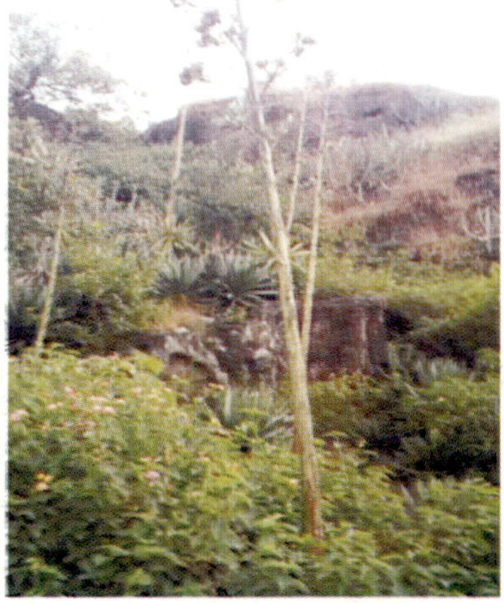

Agave americana

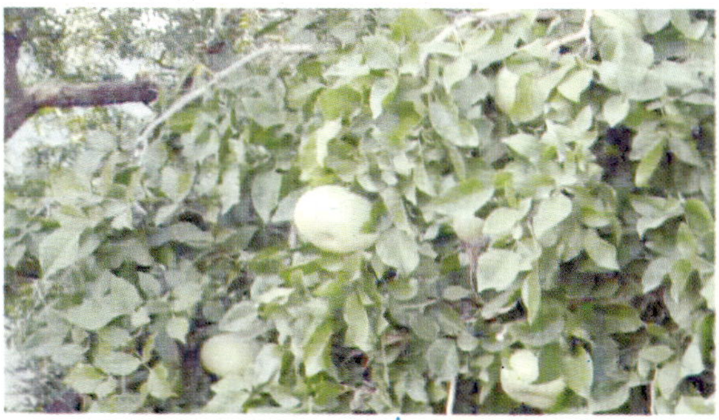

Aegle marmelos

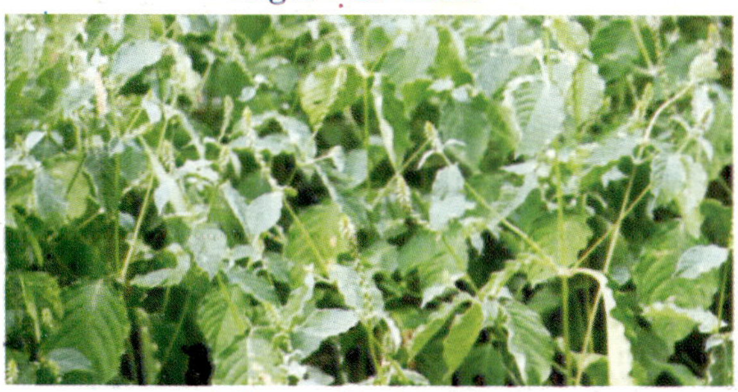

Achyranthes aspera

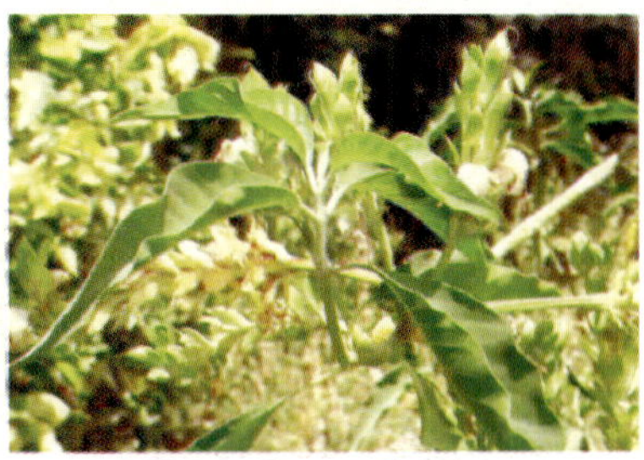

Adhatoda zeylanica

Plate - 2

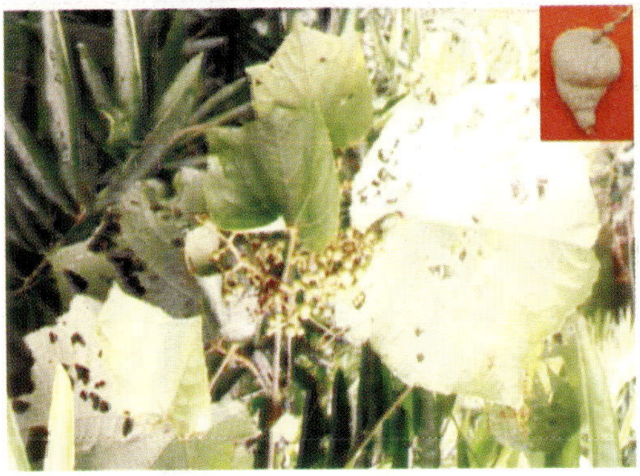

Ampelocissus latifolia

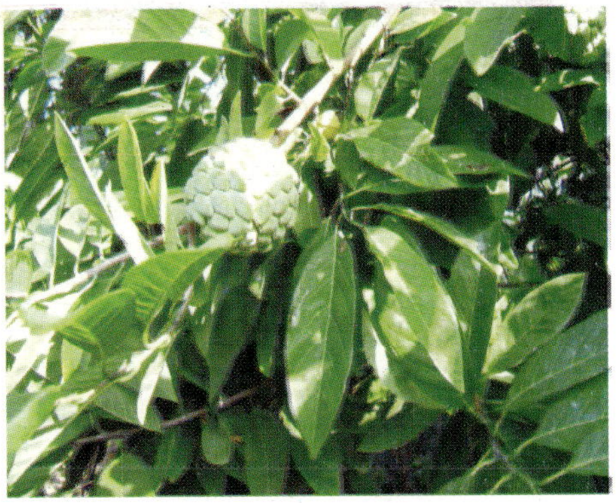

Annona squamosa

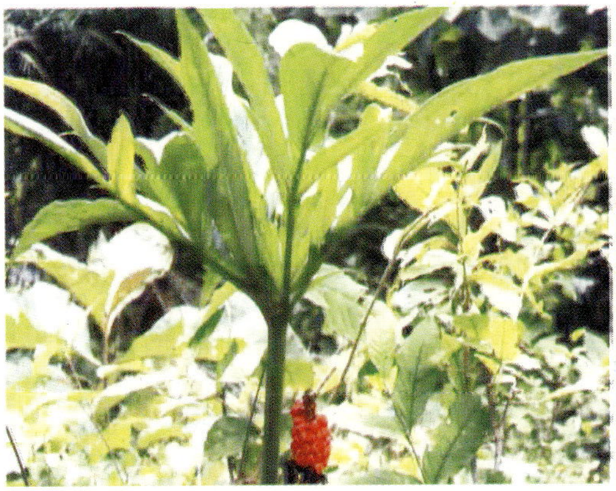

Arisaema tortuosum

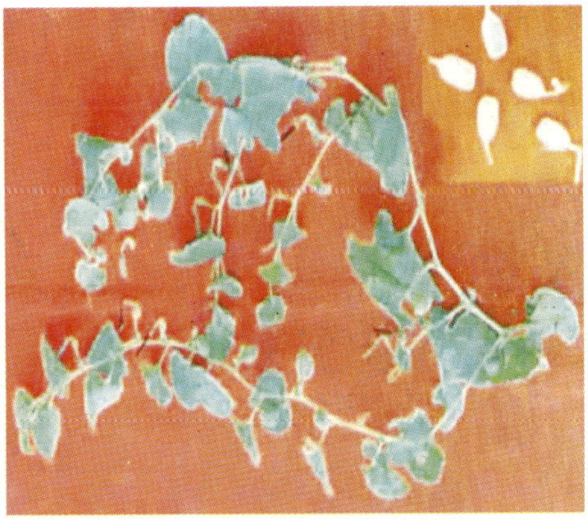

Aristolochia bracteolata

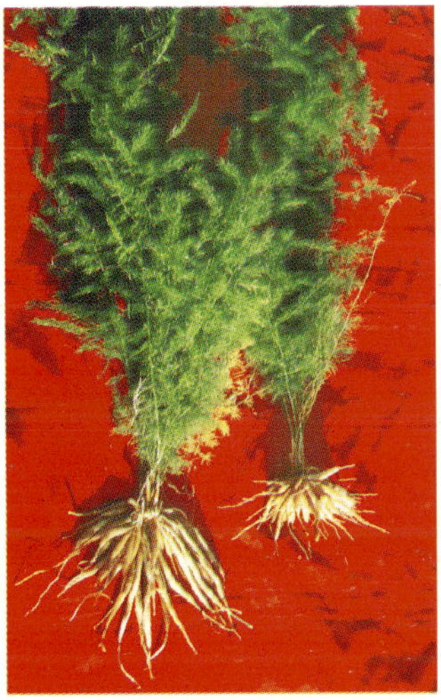

Asparagus racemosus

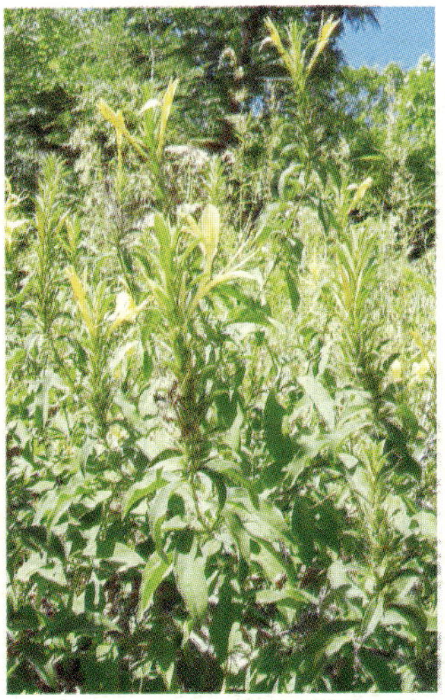

Barleria prionitis

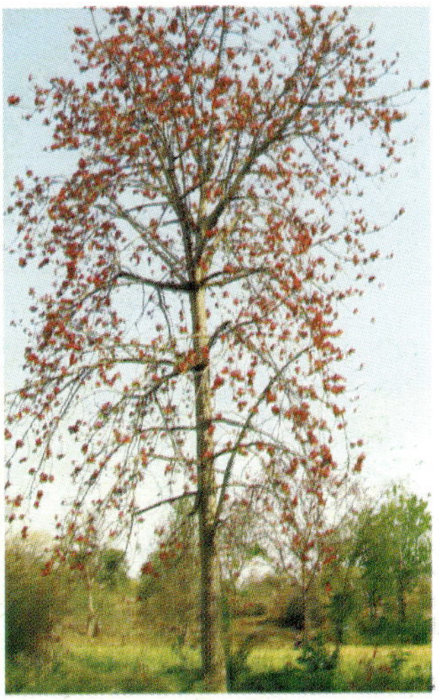

Bombax ceiba

Plate - 3

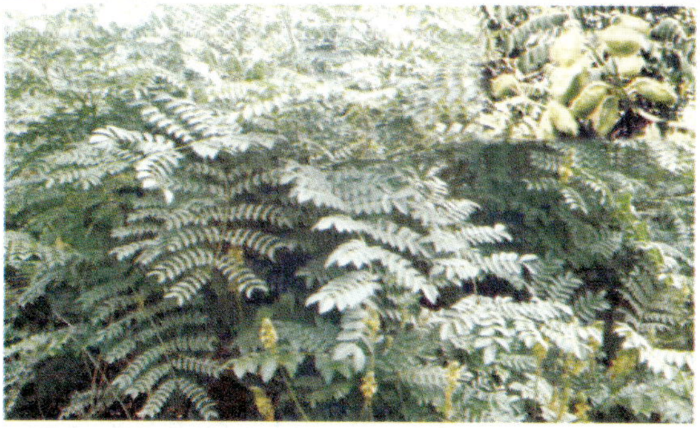

Caesalpinia bonduc

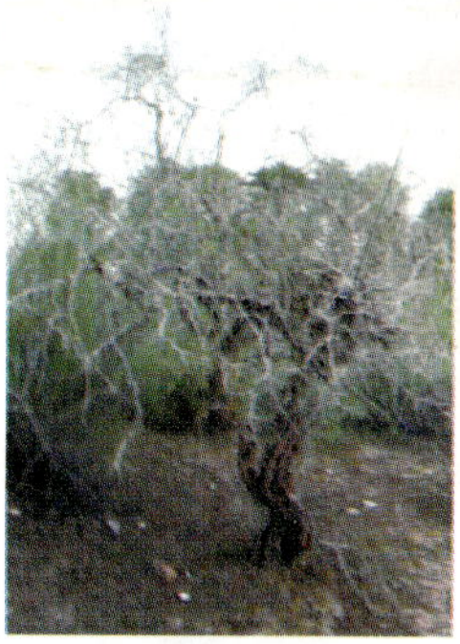

Calligonum polygonoides

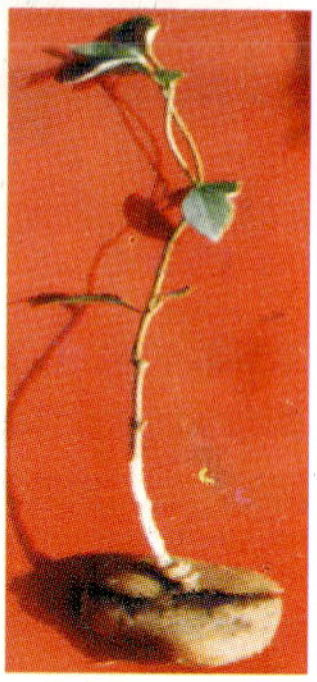

Ceropegia bulbosa

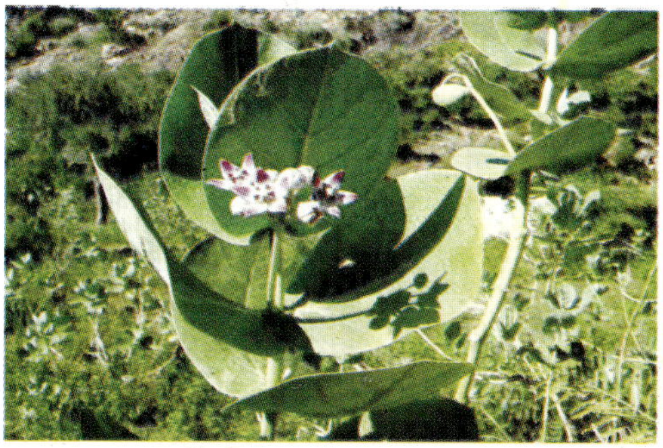

Calotropis procera

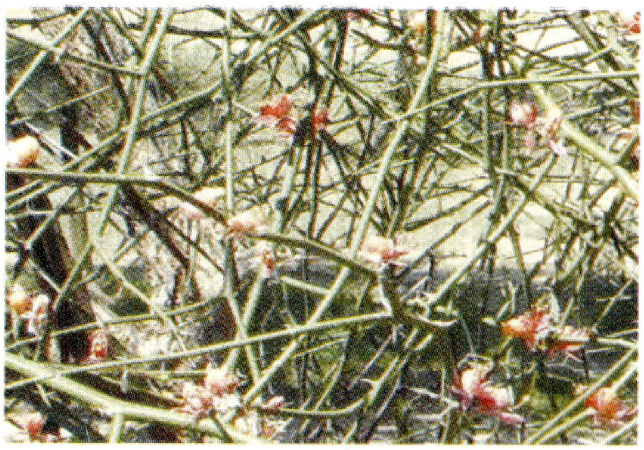

Capparis decidua

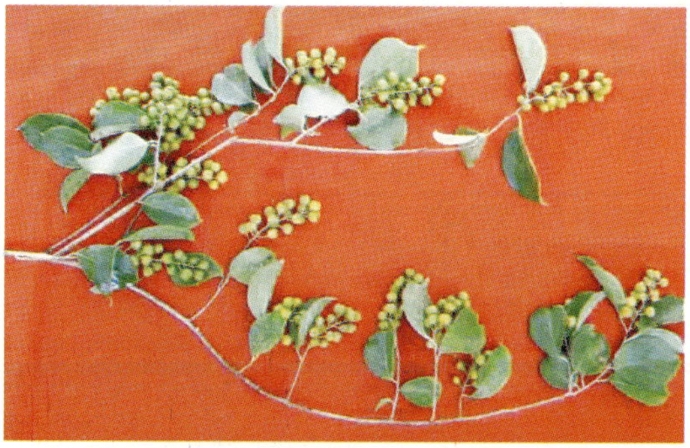

Celastrus paniculata

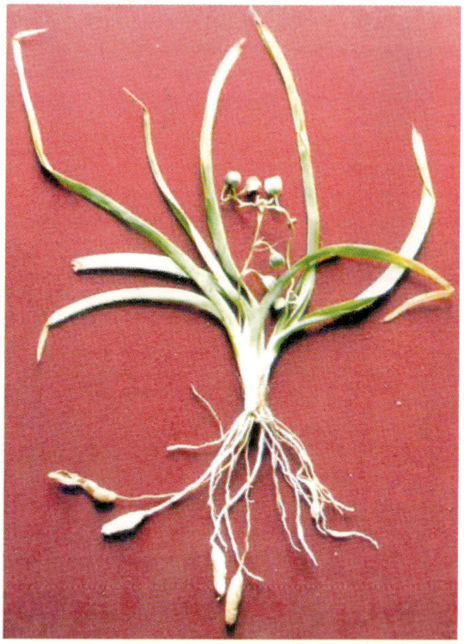

Chlorophytum tuberosum

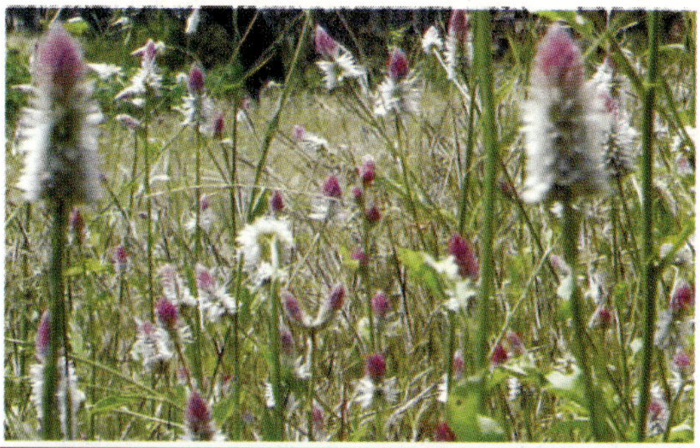

Celosia argentea

Plate - 4

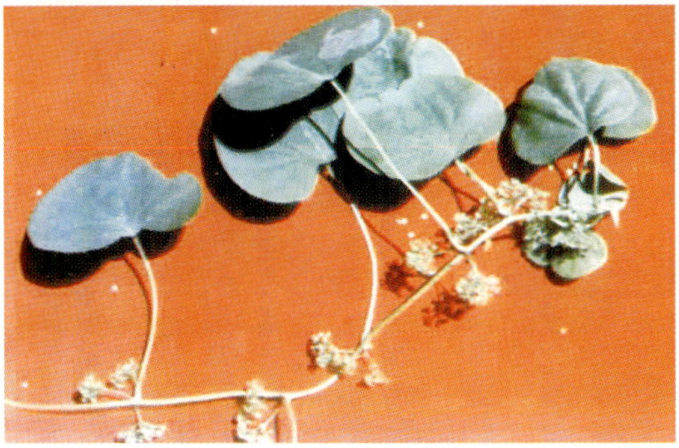

Cissampelos pareira

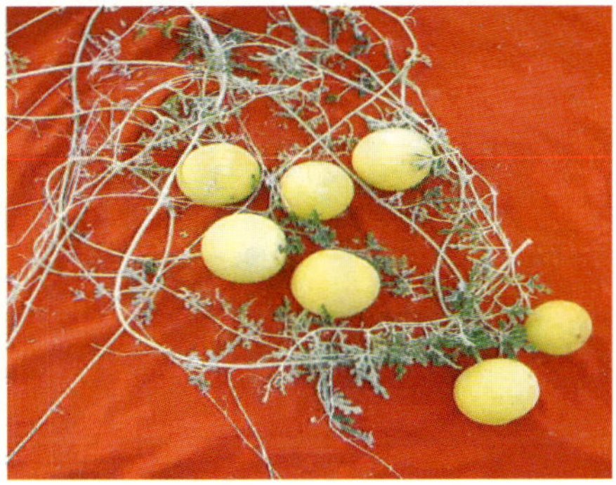

Citrullus colocynthis

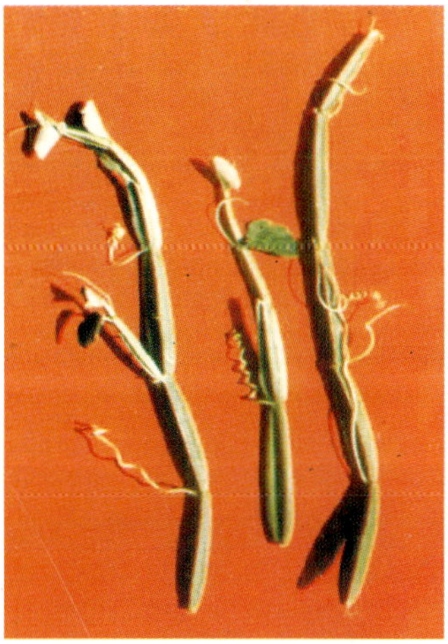

Cissus quadrangula

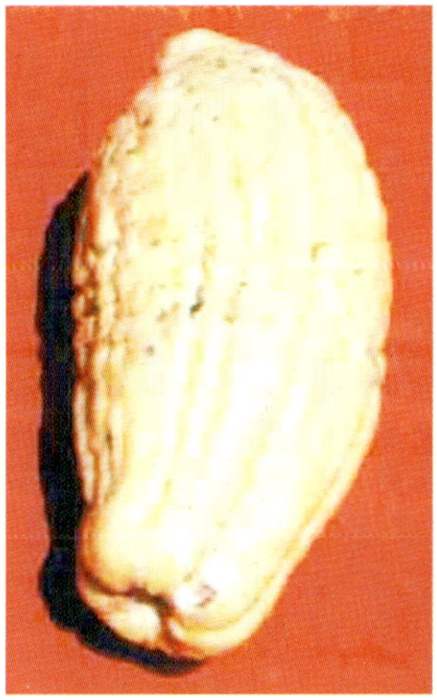

Citrus medica

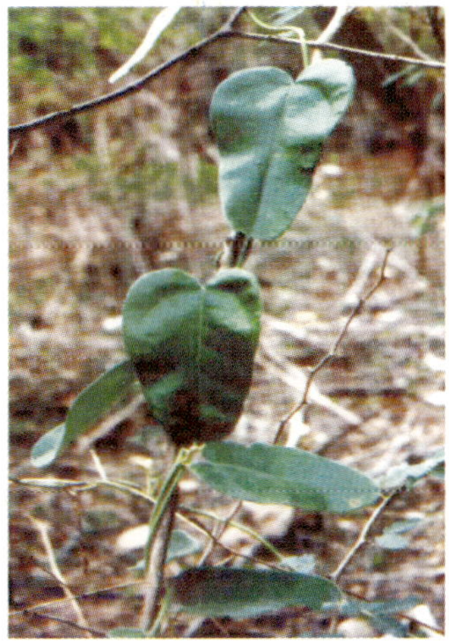

Cocculus hirsutus

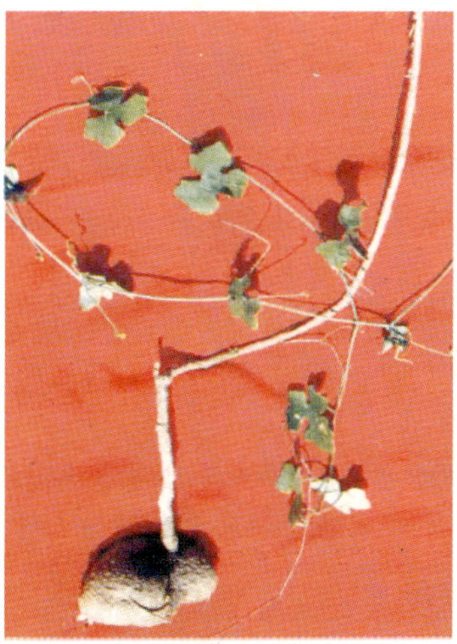

Corallocarpus epigaeus

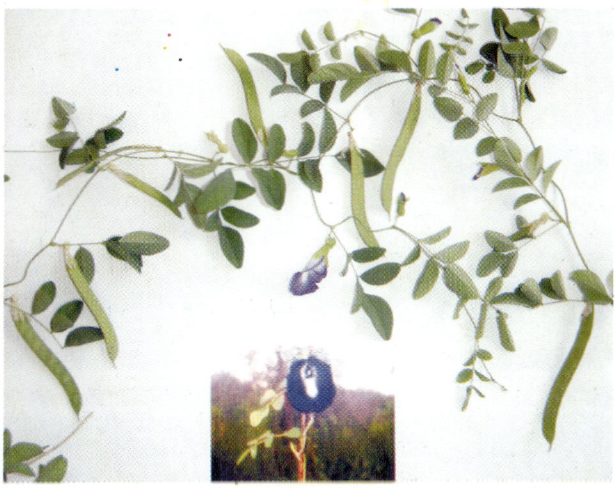

Clitoria ternatea

Plate - 5

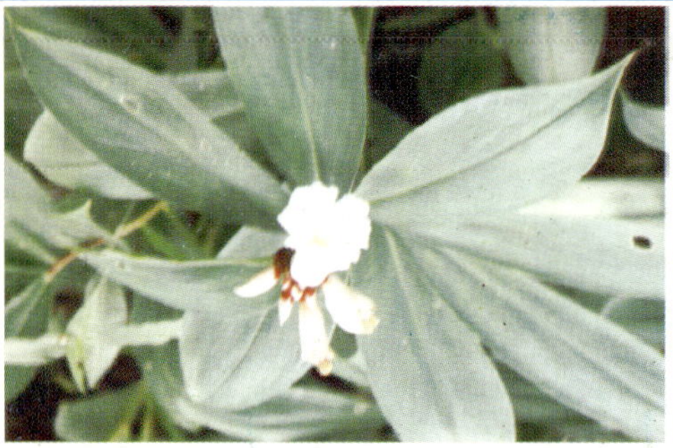

Costus speciosus

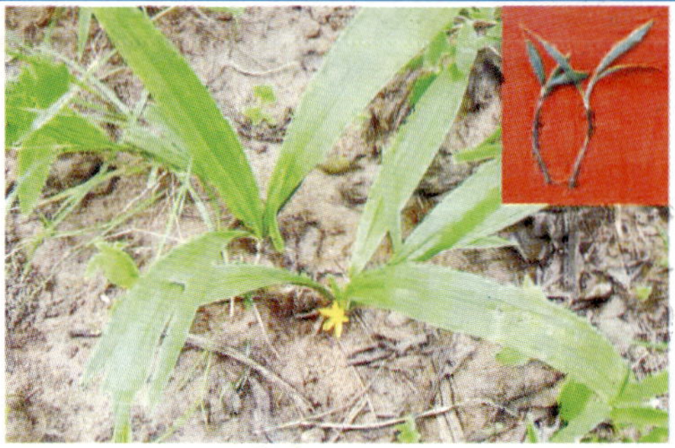

Curculigo orchioides

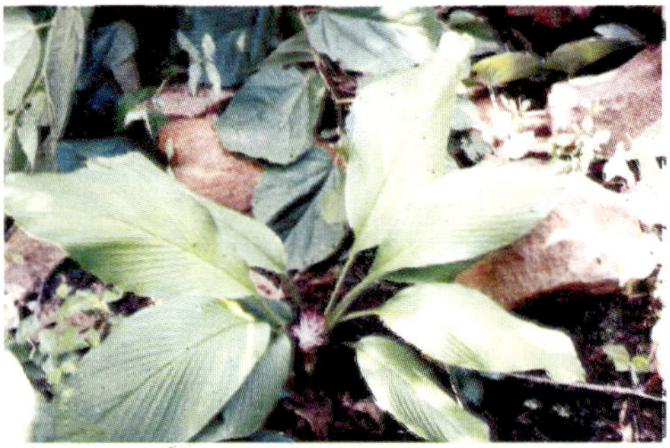

Curcuma amada

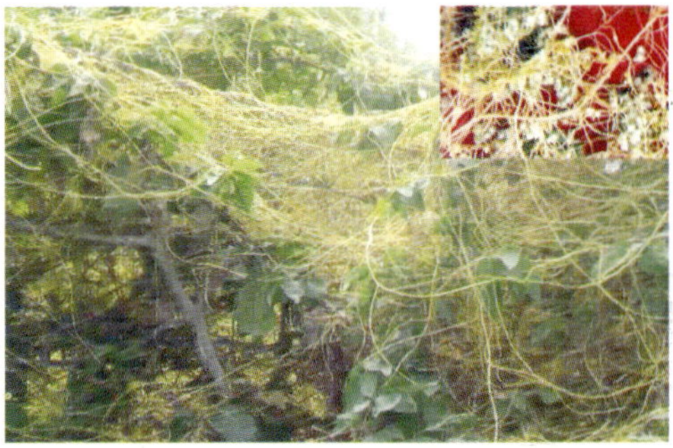

Cuscuta reflexa

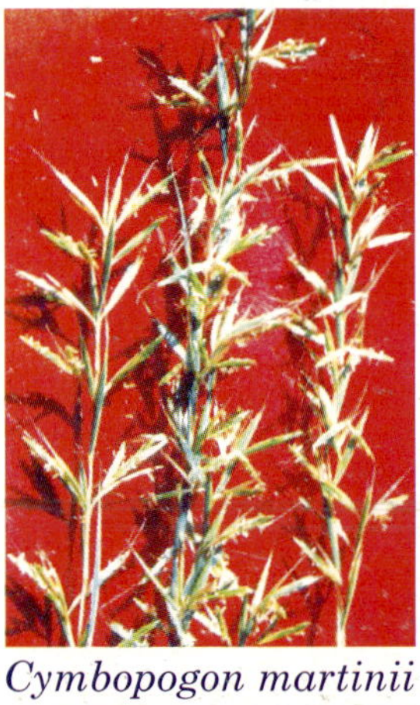

Cymbopogon martinii

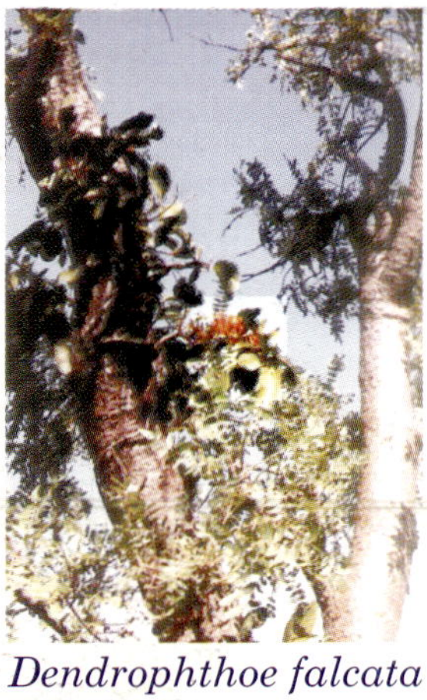

Dendrophthoe falcata

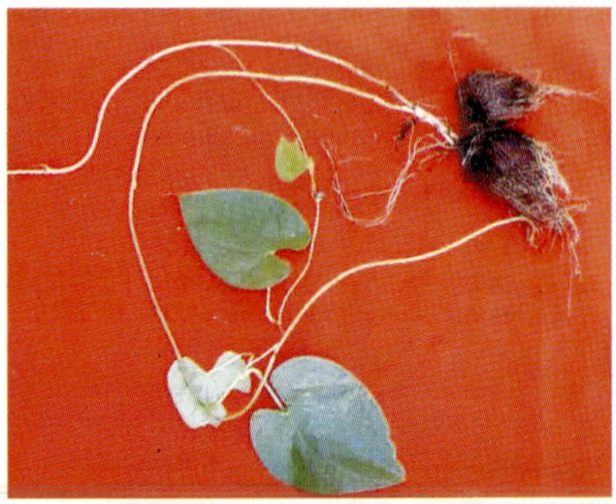

Dioscorea bulbifera

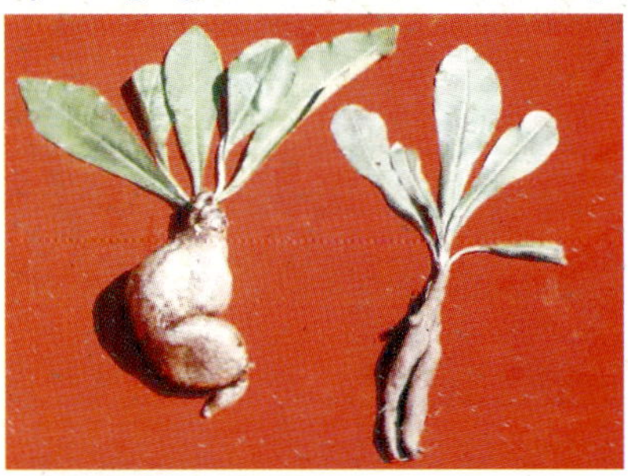

Euphorbia fusiformis

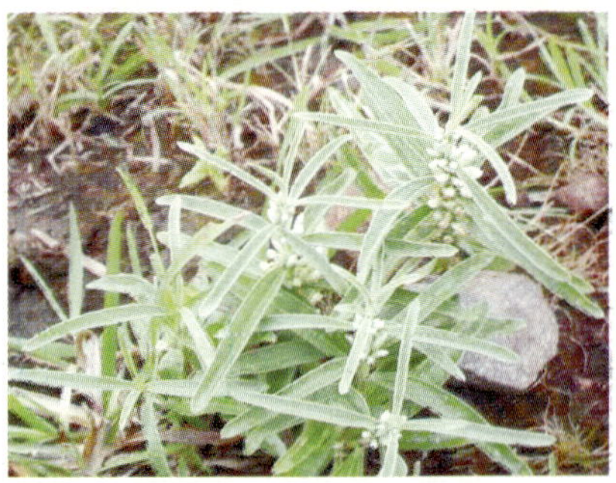

Enicostema axillare

Plate - 6

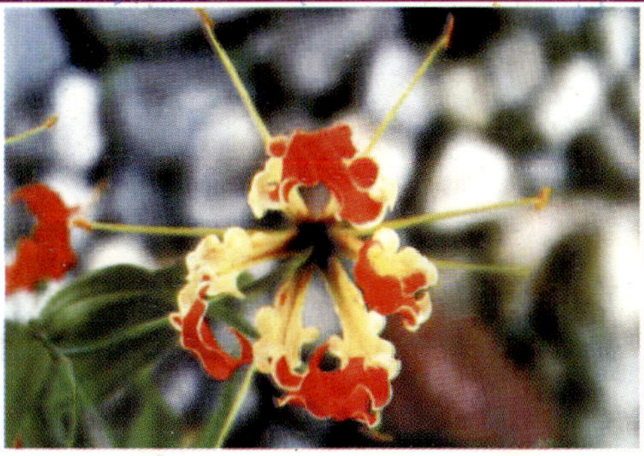

Gloriosa superba

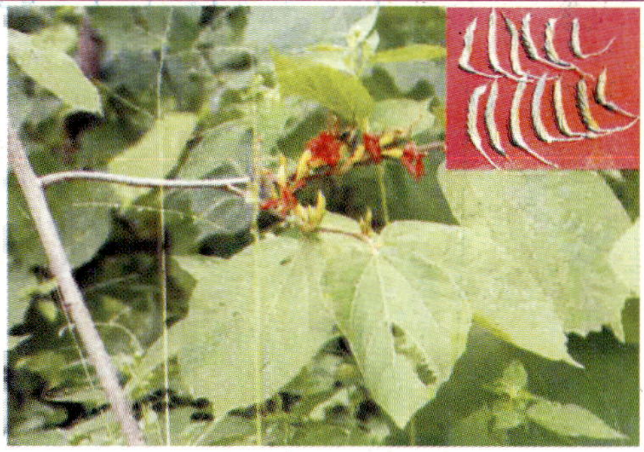

Helicteres isora

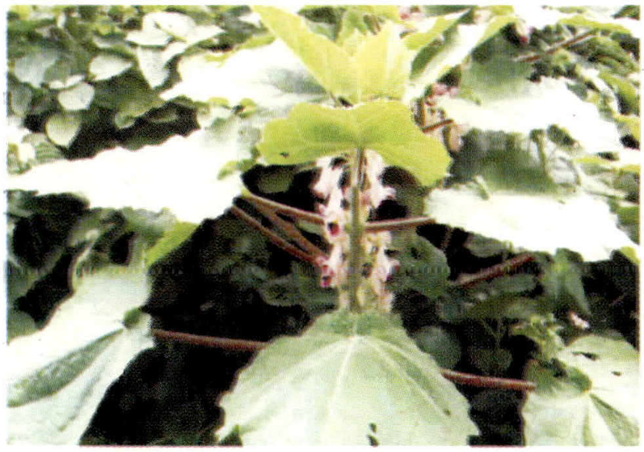

Martynia annua

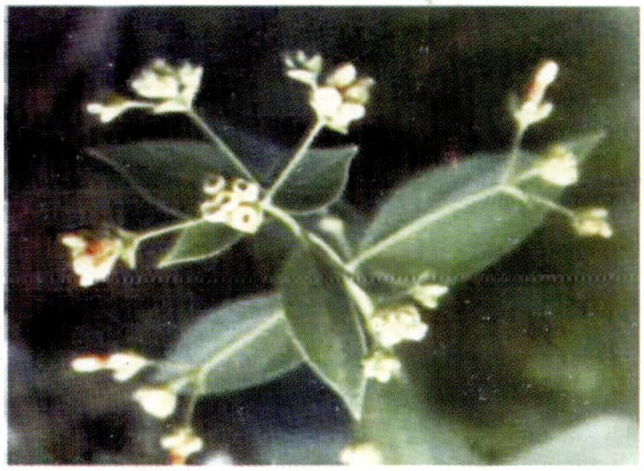

Nyctanthes arbor-tristis

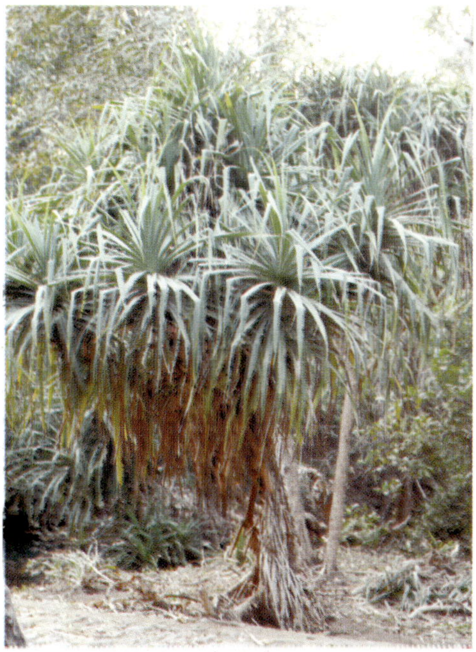

Pandanus fascicularis

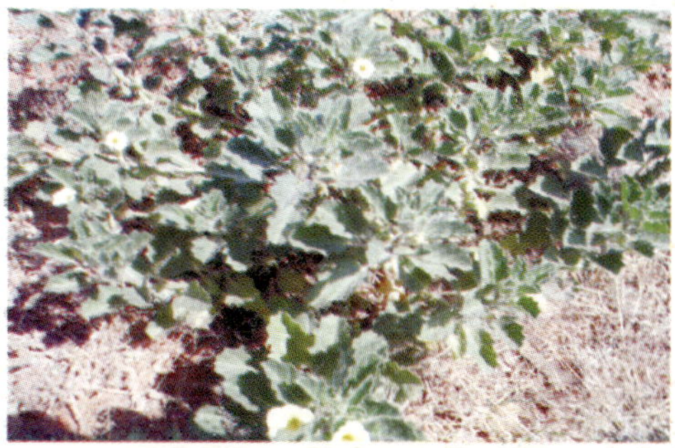

Pedalium murex

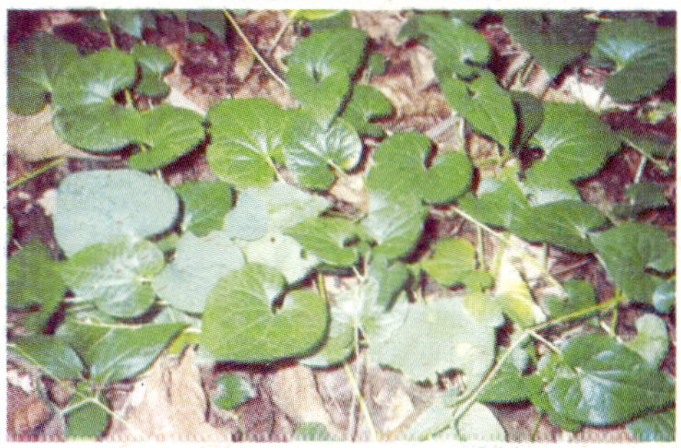

Peperomia pellucida

Plate - 7

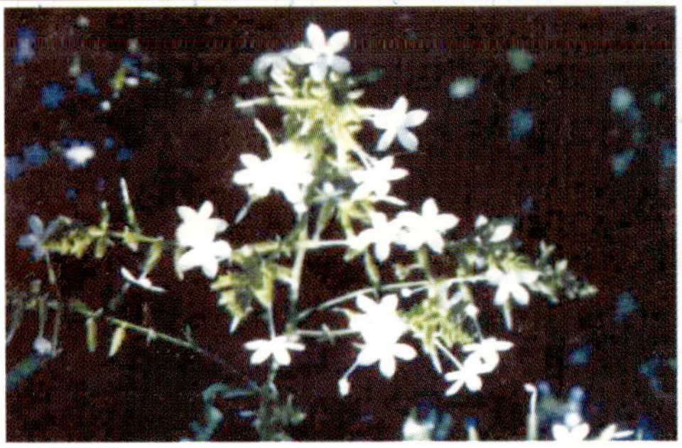

Plumbago zeylanica

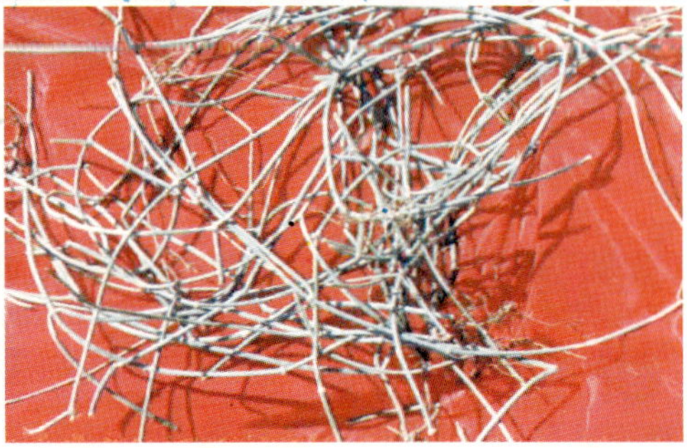

Sarcostemma viminale

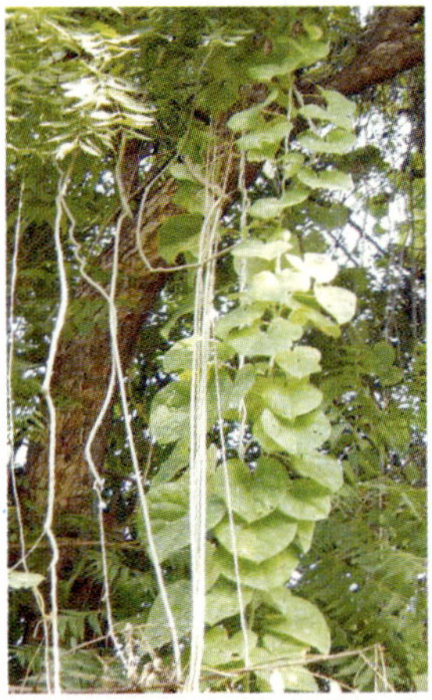

Tinospora cordifolia

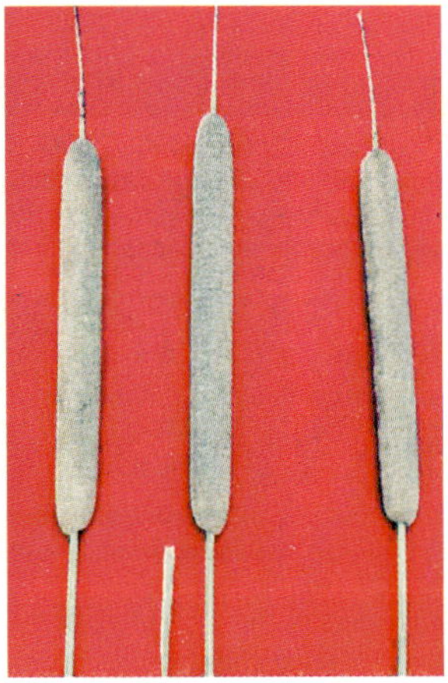

Typha angustata

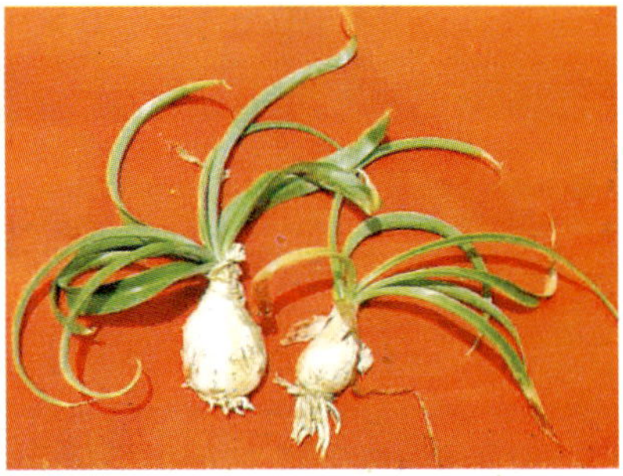

Urginea indica

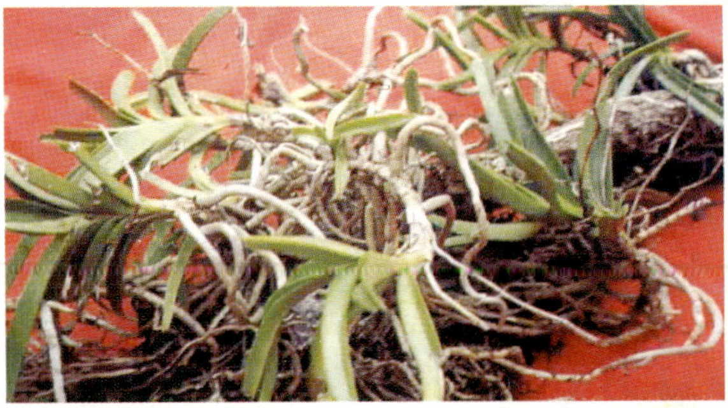

Vanda tessellata

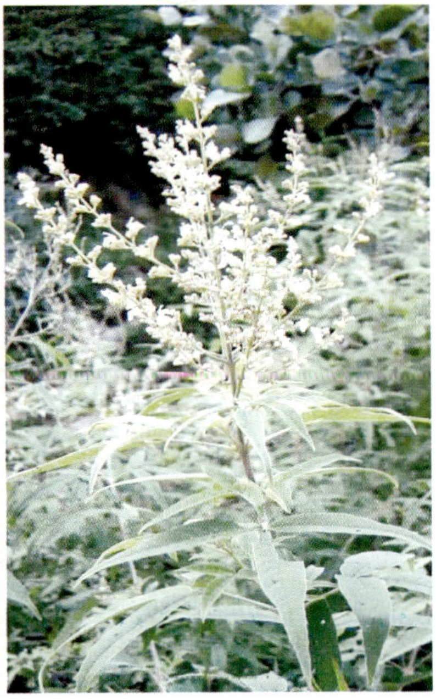

Vitex negundo

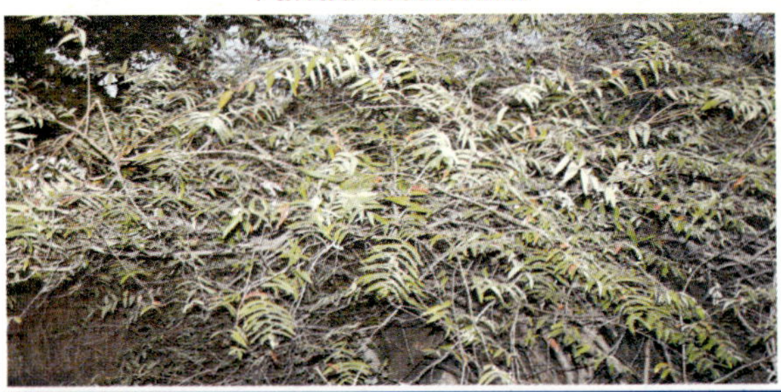

Woodfordia fruticosa

Plate - 8

Chapter 1

INTRODUCTION

Evolution of human life and culture has directly or indirectly been associated with and influenced by the surrounding environment. Primitive people live closely associated with nature and chiefly depend on it for their survival. Their dependence on plants around them made them acquire the knowledge of economic and medicinal properties of many plants by trial and error method. Consequently they became the store-house of knowledge of many useful as well as harmful plants, accumulated and enriched through generation and passed on from one generation to another, without any written document. About 75%-90% of the rural population in the world still relies on herbal medicine for their health care. The long tradition of herbal medicine continues to the present day in China, India, and many countries in Africa and South America. In many village market places, medicinal herbs are sold alongside vegetables and other wares. Practitioners of herbal medicine often undergo a rigorous and extended training to learn the names, uses, and preparation of native plants

Since the domestication of animals some 10,000 years ago, rural communities have been experimenting with and developing their own veterinary theories and techniques. The oldest known veterinary texts originate from Egypt, India and China documented as early as 269 BC. Until the early 1900's most veterinary practices could be considered traditional in the sense that they derived from long experience and underwent little fundamental change in many of their tools and techniques. With the discovery of modern chemo-therapeutics in the twentieth century, however, the First World began to abandon much of its own medical and veterinary tradition in favor of what is now viewed as conventional or modern medicine (Mc Corkle *et. al.,* 1996).

What is Ethnoveterinary Medicine?

Ethnoveterinary medicine refers to people's knowledge, skills, methods, practices and beliefs about the care of their animals (McCorkle, 1986). These traditional animal healthcare practices provide low cost alternatives in situations where western system of medicine and veterinary services are not available or are too expensive. These practices were developed and practiced through trial and error methods and deliberate experimentation and is therefore, less documented and not universally recognized and for these reasons, it has had no place in mainstream veterinary medicine.

The discovery of uses of ethnoveterinary medicinal plants must have occurred in a number of ways, not only by the principal of trial and error mechanism but also through other ways which includes; watching animals treating themselves by eating and rubbing with special plants when ill and subsequent adoption of the same remedies, communicating and interacting with other traditional ethnoveterinary medical practitioners etc. The storage of the knowledge is solely depended on the collective memory of just a few entrusted persons within communities for it is just not common knowledge for everybody. The knowledge is believed to be collectively owned by ancestors and kept under the custody of living old men and women, depending on the community, ethnicity, sex, age, caste etc. There is a danger however, this method of vesting knowledge in human custodians can be undermined by mortality, thereby losing important information to the future generations. Since the domestication of animals, livestock owners have been concerned about the health of their animals. Civilizations all over the world had their herbal experts or doctors, being the local equivalents of trained doctors, who could help their fellows in adversities. In countries like China, India, Germany etc. manufacturing of herbal remedies or phytopharmaceuticals have evolved a long way with other traditional healthcare practices and even the products are sold in country and exported.

Historically both human and animal medicine has relied heavily on traditional treatments and plant materials. The traditional theories or indigenous knowledge which is local knowledge unique to a given culture or society still forms the basis for agriculture, health care, food preparation, education, environmental conservation and a host of other activities. It is build upon and passed down from generation to generation, usually by word of mouth. Farmers and livestock raisers throughout the developing world rely on traditional practices to keep their animals healthy. Such ethnoveterinary medicine includes the use of medicinal plants, surgical techniques and management practices to prevent and treat livestock diseases. Interest in ethnoveterinary medicine has risen over the last decade. Some scientists and development professionals recognize its potential as an alternative or complement to Western-style veterinary medicine (McCorkle *et al.*, 1996).

Still the development in ethnoveterinary research is very young. Field research has mainly been done in Africa, less in Asia and very little in Latin America and elsewhere. These researches are mainly descriptive (practices, prescriptions, linguistic analyses). In the 1980s the term "Veterinary Anthropology" was coined for a particular approach to animal health care, which was researched through "using the basic repertoire of anthropology's research skills and techniques, including observation, interview and participation" (Köhler-Rollefson and Bräunig, 1998).

Ethnoveterinary information is in danger of extinction because of the current rapid changes in communities all over the world. In fact, many communities nowadays use a mix of local and modern practices. Promoting the conservation and use of ethnoveterinary medicine does not mean downgrading or ignoring the value of modern medicine and attempting to replace one with the other. However, it does mean recognizing that both types have their strengths and limitations. In some instances, they complement each other, in others, local practices will be the better choice, and again in others modern practices should be recommended.

Aspects of Ethnoveterinary medicine

Ethnoveterinary medicine is often taken to mean using medicinal herbs. However, it has more to offer:

Information: Stock raisers commonly know when their animals are sick. They can describe the disease signs, which season the disease commonly strikes, and what types of animals are affected. They also know where to find the best pasture, how to avoid tsetse-infested areas, where to find saltlicks, and many, many other things.

Practices: This is much wider than just the use of herbal medicines. It also covers bone-setting, vaccination against pox and other infectious diseases, branding, and careful management practices.

Beliefs: Beliefs are commonly thought of as superstitious - something negative that has to be suppressed. Still, some beliefs can be very useful because they improve the animals' condition or prevent them from getting sick. Examples are the feeding of salt that has been blessed, protecting animals against evil winds, and not letting animals on pastures where other animals have died from diseases such as anthrax. So it is advisable to have a close look at beliefs and encourage these if they promote animal health.

Breeds: Local breeds, such as dairy buffaloes, are the outcome of centuries of selection. At first sight, they may produce less than introduced breeds, but they may not score as poorly if both input costs and outputs are considered, instead of only the outputs. Local breeds are presently receiving increased attention in connection with attempts to conserve their dwindling genetic resources.

Human resources: Knowledgeable farmers, herders and local healers are treasurers of knowledge and can be valuable partners in development projects.

Ethnoveterinary versus modern medicine

Farmers in West Java, Indonesia, raise their goats and sheep in sheds on stilts with a slatted floor, and feed them with cut fodder. As a result the animals have few intestinal worms. If an animal gets ill, the farmer drenches it with a preparation of herbs using recipes learned from her parents or husband.

While West Javanese smallholders commonly boil parts from several herbs, Samburu pastoralists in Kenya often make medicines by soaking just one plant. These are only two examples of the many ways livestock raisers all over the world keep their animals healthy and productive. 'Ethnoveterinary medicine' contrasts the knowledge developed by local livestock holders from the scientific or 'allopathic' veterinary medicine taught at universities. Both are dynamic and changing. Like scientific veterinary medicine, ethnoveterinary practices have been developed through trial-and-error and deliberate experimentation. But ethnoveterinary medicine is developed by farmers in fields and barns, rather than by scientists in laboratories and clinics. It is less systematic and less formalized, and is usually transferred by word of mouth rather than in writing.

Ethnoveterinary medicine differs not only from region to region but also among and within communities. Depending on the work division and professional specialization, men may know more about large animals while women commonly are more familiar with small animals or with certain type of diseases such as mastitis and neonatal care. Hunters may have a wealth of information on hunting dogs. Knowing about such differences can be crucial in the selection of respondents in research and partners for extension approaches, the design of training courses, and the selection of trainees for community-based animal health workers.

In India, enough attention has not yet been given to the traditional veterinary herbal remedies. Even the 'Regveda', Athrvaveda' and eight divisions of 'Ayurveda' the pioneer documents with curative properties of plants, have not provided much information on veterinary remedies (Pal, 1984). There has been a rich tradition and indigenous knowledge about animal healthcare in India. However, during the last hundred years or so, there has been a decline in the practice of Ayurveda and Unani system of veterinary medicine in preference to western veterinary practice based on chemical and synthetic drugs. In rural areas, remedies based on locally available herbs are still prevalent. Modern health care in the tribal and rural areas is characterized by the deficiency of infrastructure, of qualified personnel and of medicine. Access to and within the region is extremely difficult during certain periods of the year making evacuation for medicinal treatment an unrealistic alternative. Given these extreme conditions, the population has recourse almost solely to traditional medicine.

Recently, the first online Ethnoveterinary data bank and an international mailing list have been developed (International Network Prelude, 2002). On the other hand, interdisciplinary field studies focused on traditional knowledge related to veterinary practices have rarely been conducted, and most have been focused mainly on the description of animal health management practices and much less on the bioscientific and anthropological evaluation of traditional remedies. Systemic Ethnoveterinary studies on remedies used in traditional phototherapeutic practices have been carried out mainly in Africa, Asia and Central America (Lans *et al,* 2000, 2001; Scarpa, 2000; Nfi *et al.*, 2001; Alawa *et al.*, 2002; Ole-Miaron, 2003). In Europe, medicinal plants used in folk veterinary practices have been specifically investigated in only a few field studies (Blanca *et al.*, 1999; Uncini Manganelli *et al.,* 2001; Waller *et al.*, 2001; Pieroni *et al.*, 2004).

From analysis of literature on ethnoveterinary medicine some conclusions can be drawn. Ethnoveterinary research and development is still very young, field research has mainly been done in Africa, less in Asia and very little in Latin America and elsewhere. These researches are mainly descriptive (practices, prescriptions, linguistic analyses). Few analytical studies (e.g. Bachmann, 1998; compared the knowledge of pastoralists with epidemiological data on contagious *caprine pleuropneumonia*) have been carried out (Mathias, 1996). Major work in this field has been done by women (Evelyn Matthias and Constance McCorkle especially), a veterinarian and a sociologist, a combination which has led to a broader understanding (Van't Hooft, 1995).

India is now beginning to search her roots in the past and revive her lost glory of the traditional system of medicine which flourished here for several centuries and contributed much to the development of the medical science of world. To alleviate the sufferings of her large ever growing populace, she has to revive the Traditional Folklore Medicine and bring it into the mainstream of National Health-Care Program. An account of botanical ethnoveterinary prescriptions in India and Rajasthan has been given by Sebastian and Bhandari, 1984; Reddy and Sudarshan, 1987; Jain, 1991, 1999; Livestock Census, 2003; Sharma, 2005; Sikarwar *et al.* 1994; Joshi, 1995; Dwivedi, 1998; Singh and Pandey, 1998; Kumar, 2002, 2006; Katewa and Chaudhary, 2000; Anjaria *et al.,* 2002; Anonymous, 2004; Kumar *et al.*, 2004; Mokat and Deokule, 2004; Khoda, 2005; Swarup and Patra, 2005; Unnikrishnan and Shankar, 2005; Katewa and Jain, 2006; Kadel and Jain, 2006; Nag *et al.*, 2006, 2007; Tiwari and Pande, 2006 Yadav, 2007; Galav *et al.,* 2007, Mini and Shivdasan, 2007and Jain *et al.*, 2008.

In the present book, an attempt has been made to document the precious traditional knowledge on folklore ethnoveterinary medicines of Rajasthan, which could provide future drugs for some dreadful diseases that plague animals. Ethnoveterinary medicines are of specific value in developing countries where allopathic veterinary medicines are often beyond the reach of livestock producers. It can play an important role in grassroot development, which seeks to empower people by enhancing the use of their own knowledge and resources. The present book is also intended to contribute to this growing body of knowledge by supplying information on the plant, animal and mineral based Ethnoveterinary curative techniques found in tribal areas of Rajasthan.

Attempt has also been made to name the tribe making specific use and methods of preparation of the drug, dosage and duration have also been highlighted. The enumeration of species is made alphabetically and the name of family is given in parenthesis for easy consultation. The ethnoveterinary information has been categorized on the basis of ailments and herbs used for treatment to make the book easy to consult. The language used in the book is easily understandable, and indices to the local names and botanical names have been given at the end of book. The photographs and line diagrams of some important plants have been provided to make the book more useful.

CHAPTER 2

STUDY AREA AND METHODOLOGY

Rajasthan is the largest state of India occupying an area of 34.22 million ha., which constitutes 10.41 percent of the land area of the country. It lies between latitudes 23°3' and 30°12' north and longitudes 69°30' and 78°17' east. The state is bounded by Pakistan in the west and north-west; by the state of Punjab in the north; by Haryana in the north-east; by Uttar Pradesh in the east; by Madhya Pradesh in the south-east and Gujarat in south-west. It is one of the few states of India that show great contrast from one area to another. This disparity is noticeable in respect of climate, soil, vegetation, mineral resource etc. The state is immensely rich in natural beauty. Its beautiful forests and valleys are as famous as its desert. Geographically, no other region can claim greater diversity than Rajasthan; a region of lofty hills and rolling sand dunes, of scorching heat and freezing cold, of fertile plains in the east and sparsely populated areas of Jaisalmer in the west. The state presents a Kaleidoscope of ecosystems and divided into 32 districts, 30 Zila Parishads and 241 Tehsils. Rajasthan has a lower population density (129/km2) compared to India (274/km2) (1991) and higher percentage of rural population (71.12%) showing that the state is still predominantly rural and dependent upon agriculture as the mainstay livelihood. The state may be divided into 6 regions: (1) Western arid region (2) Semi-arid region (3) South-eastern region (4) Chambal ravines (5) Aravalli region and (6) Eastern region.

The most striking geological feature of Rajasthan is the Aravalli range the oldest mountain range in the world, which intersects the state end to end north-east to south-west diagonally, covering about 30 percent area of the state. The Aravalli mountain range that runs from Delhi to Gujarat divide the state into two unequal halves. The north-west region covering two thirds (61 per cent of the total area) and 11 districts of the state falls under the Thar desert, which is dry and arid region consisting mostly of a series of sand dunes. The eastern region has large fertile tracts. The forest of Sariska, Ranthambhor, Raolitatgarh, Kumbhalgarh and Mount Abu are situated in the Aravallis. Aravallis highest peak is Gurushikhar (1727 meter) near Mount Abu. This is the mountain chain which possess great water divide of India and originates rivers, flowing both side i.e. east and west. For example, Eastern Banas, originates near Kumbhalgarh, flows eastwards and ultimately joins river Chambal near Madhya Pradesh border while Western Banas, also originates close to Kumbhalgarh, flows west wards and drains its water into Arabian Sea. The western and north western Rajasthan covering entire Jodhpur and Bikaner divisions and part of Jaipur and Ajmer divisions falls under the desert land. The Desert National Park provides ample evidence of the fact that once upon a time, this area was woodland. The western desert is characterized by arid landscape, barren hills, sandy hummocks, sandy plains and sand dunes. Rajasthan is known as "Dharti Dhoran Ri" (Land of sand dunes) owing to profusion of sand dunes in Thar Desert. The largest active dune the SAM SAND DUNE (Jaisalmer) is a recognized tourist attraction. To the south east of Aravallis fall the eastern plains consisting of the southern and eastern portions, which merge with the more equitable climatic zones of peninsular India. The eastern plains have rich alluvial soil, drained by the seasonal rivers like Banas and Mahi. The region covers mainly the area of Tonk, Ajmer, Jaipur, Dausa, Sawaimadhopur districts.

Soil plays an important role in agricultural development and planning of a region. Various type of soils are found in Rajasthan; desert soil, gypsiferrous, grey brown alluvial soil, non calcify brown soil, Alluvial soils of recent origin, hilly soil, red loam and deep medium black soil. Soil of western Rajasthan is desertic type and contains 90 to 95 per cent sand and about 5 to 7 per cent clay. Water is scarce in this type of soil.

The climate of the state varies from semi-arid to arid. Marked variations in diurnal and seasonal range of temperature occur at all places in the state, exhibiting the most characteristic phenomenon of the warm-dry continental climate. The isotherms of summer (June) show variations from 42°C (Sirohi district) to above 47°C (Ganganagar district). A major part of the state, comprising the arid zone of the west and the semi-arid zone of the mid-west, has an average maximum of 45°C in this month. However, in the south-eastern parts, the isotherms show a declining trend from 43°C to 37°C. The isotherms of winter (January), ranging from less than 6°C in the north to above 10°C in the south-east, show few variations in temperature. The greater part of Rajasthan, except the south-eastern part of Kota, Bundi and Baran and the western district of Barmer exhibits the mean temperature of more than 10°C. The secondary depressions (western disturbances) accompanied by the ice-cold winds, emanating from the higher latitudes may bring entire Rajasthan under the spell of the cold wave for the periods of 2 to 5 days during winter months.

To the west of the Aravalli range the climate is characterized by low rainfall with erratic distribution, extremes of diurnal and annual temperature, low humidity and high wind veloc1ty. The climate is semi-arid to sub-humid in the east of the Aravalli range, characterized by more or less the same extremes in temperature but relatively lower wind velocity and high humidity with better rainfall. The entire state is characterized by hyperthermic conditions. The annual rainfall in the state varies significantly. The general trend of isohyets is from north-west to south-east. There is a very rapid and marked decrease in rainfall west of the Aravalli range making western Rajasthan the most arid part. The average annual rainfall in this part ranges from less than 10 cm in north-west part of Jaisalmer (lowest in the state), to 20 to 30 cm in Ganganagar, Bikaner and Barmer regions, 30 to 40 cm in Nagaur, Jodhpur, Churu and Jalore regions and more than 40 cm in Sikar, Jhunjhunu and Pali regions and along the western fringes of the Aravalli range. On the eastern side of the Aravalli range, the rainfall ranges from 55 cm in Ajmer to 102 cm in Jhalawar. In plains, Banswara (92.0 cm) and Jhalawar (95 cm) districts receive the maximum annual rain. Mount Abu (Sirohi district) in the south-west, however, receives the highest rainfall in the state (163.8 cm). The yearly total rainfall is highly variable at different places all over the state and it is most erratic in the western half with frequent spells of drought, punctuated occasionally by heavy downpour in some years, associated with the passing low pressure systems over the region.

There are two forest type namely Tropical Dry Deciduous and Tropical Thorn forest. Forests are mostly confined in eastern and southern parts of the state. The western part of the state is devoid of forest because of prevailing hot arid condition. The total forest area is 3.17 million ha which constitutes 9.26% of geographical area of the state. By legal status, reserved forest constitutes 37%, protected forest 53% and unclassed forest 10 per cent. In the protected area there are 4 national parks and 24 wildlife sanctuaries, covering an area of 0.96 million ha, which constitutes 2.8% of the geographical area of the state. Ranthambhor and Sariska are the two tiger reserve located in the state. Keoladeo Ghana national park, Bharatpur is of internat-ional importance for its rich avifauna and for migratory Siberian crane. There are 37,889 villages in the state of which 7,114 have forests as a land use. In these villages, about 2.11 million ha is classified as forest. The total population of these villages is 6.78

million. The villages having less than 100 ha, between 100-500 ha and more than 5000 ha forest in each village constitutes 47 per cent, 39 per cent and 14% of the total villages respectively (Census, 1991). The forest cover of the state, based on satellite data of October-December, 1996, is 13871 sq. km. which is 4.03 of the geographical area. Dense and open forest account for 4,309 sq. Km and 9,562 sq. Km, respectively.

Tribes of Rajasthan

Rajasthan's population includes many tribals, who today constitute 12% of the state population, nearly double the national average. The main tribes of Rajasthan are the Bhils and the Minas that were the original inhabitants of the area now called Rajasthan. But they were forced into the Aravalli range by the Aryan invasion. Smaller tribes include the Sahariyas, Garasias and the Gaduliya lohars.

The tribes share common traits, which seem to link their past together but it is the differences in their costumes and jewellery, fair and festivals that set them apart from one another.

Bhils

The Bhils comprises 39.5% of Rajasthan's tribal population. Their stronghold is Banswara. The generic term derives from Bhils, which describe their original talent and strength. The Bhils maintained their numbers by mingling with rebellious outcaste Rajputs. According to legends, the Bhils were fine archers. Bhil bowmen are mentioned in both the Mahabarata and Ramayan. They were highly regarded as warriors and the Rajput rulers relied on them. Although originally food gatherers, the Bhils these days have taken up small-scale agriculture, city residence and employment.

The Baneshwar fair is a Bhil festival held near Dungarpur in January/February each year and large number of Bhils gather for several days for singing, dancing and worshipping. Holi is another important time for Bhils. Witchcraft magic and superstition are deeply rooted aspects of the Bhil culture.

Minas

The Minas are the largest and comprises 53.5% of total tribal population of the state and are the most widely spread. They may have been original inhabitants of the Indus Valley civilization. The Vedas and the Mahabharta mention them, and it was the Kachhawah Rajputs who finally dispersed them and forced them into the

Aravallis. The Minas have a tall, athletic build with sharp features, large eyes, thick lips and a light brown complexion. They live in the regions of Shekhawati and eastern Rajasthan. The name Minas is derived from `men fish'. Originally they were a ruling tribe, but their slow downfall began with the Rajputs, and was completed when the British Government declared them a 'Criminal tribe' in 1924, mainly to stop them from trying to regain their territory from the Rajputs. Just like the Bhils, the literacy rate among the Minas was very low, but is improving. Marriage, arranged by the parents is generally within the tribe and most marriages take place when the children are quite young.

Gaduliya Lohars

The Gaduliya Lohars, named after their beautiful bullock carts (`gadis'), were originally a martial Rajput tribe, but now a days they are nomadic blacksmiths. They are said to have wandered from their homeland of Mewar because of their promise to their 'lord' Maharana Pratap who was ousted from Chittorgarh by Akbar. This clan of warring Rajputs vowed to re-enter the city only after the victory of Maharana Pratap who was, however, unfortunately killed in the battlefield.

Garasias

They are a small Rajput tribe found along the Abu Road area of Southern Rajasthan. The Garasias have an interesting custom of marriage through elopement, which usually takes place at the annual Gaur fair held during the full moon in March. After the elopement, which can be spontaneous or pre- arranged, a bride price is paid to the bride's father.

Sahariyas

They are thought to be of Bhil origin and are found in the areas of Kota, Dungarpur and Sawai Madhopur in the south-east of the state. The Sahariyas are jungle dwellers, their name possibly deriving from the Persian 'Sehr'. The Sahariyas are regarded as the most backward tribe in Rajasthan and make out a living as shifting cultivators and by hunting and fishing.

Damors

The small tribal community of Damors probably migrated from their original home in Gujarat to settle in Dungarpur and Udaipur districts. They are mainly cultivators and manual labourers.

METHODOLOGY

Collection of Ethnoveterinary medicinal information

Ethnoveterinary medicinal surveys were conducted repeatedly by the authors in different seasons and areas of the state of Rajasthan for the last 10 years or so. The traditional knowledge of plant based remedies for the treatment of ailments rests with the medicinemen, all of which belong to one family of hereditary indigenous practitioners. Skills and experience are passed on from one generation to the next by word of mouth and are guarded like secrets. The medicinemen collects the plants needed for a particular application, either directly from the forest or farm or from the local shops. A number of elderly people were interviewed who have a great deal of practical knowledge about the plants, animals and minerals used as veterinary medicines in the native system.

Before actually launching into the fieldwork, rapport was established with one or two persons preferably the chief, guidance sought and contact was then established with other tribals of the locality. The linguistic fluency, personality and social standing are crucial to establishrapport between the participants involved. Field sites were visited with the local medicinemen. Generally, the informant do not want to give all the information about plants and animals. For this reason selection of informants is an important aspect of ethnobotanical study in the field. Experienced people, such as some elders, healers, medicinemen, birth- attendant, woodcutter, shepherds, headmen and Bhopa (village priest) can provide important information on useful plants, animals and minerals (Plate 1). A discussion about a particular herb with different informants from different places tends to be more helpful to record various queries about the herbal drug. Also, personal observations are helpful for verification of the data provided by the informants at different places.

To determine the authenticity of information collected during fieldwork, repeated verification of data from different people and at different times was done. Thus, only the specific and reliable information cross-checked with many informant has been incorporated in the present study.

Identification, collection and preparation of medicinal plants

Identification

The local names of plants vary from one place to another. Different plant species may have the same local name. The botanical name of each plant used in this book is given with each remedy. Before using the plant following things should be checked:

Type of plant

- Approximate size of the plant.
- Type: tree, woody, shrub, climber, grass.
- The position of flower or fruit in the plant (such as on the top of stem or in the branches).

Leaves

- Approximate size
- Shape (number of leaflets or lobes, with ridges or not) and colour.
- Texture (smooth or rough, with hair or not).
- Position and arrangement of the leaves

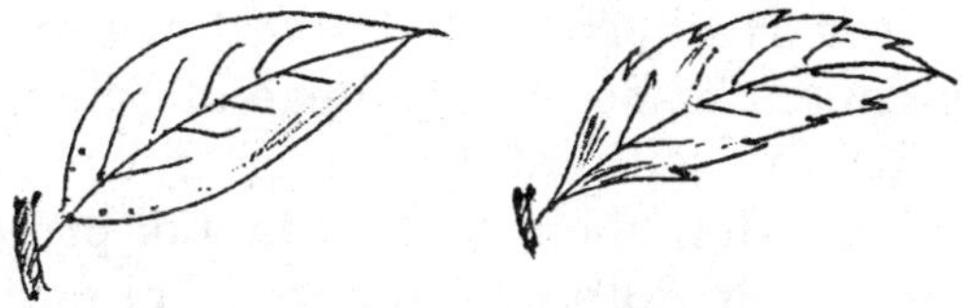

Leaves

Flowers

- Type of flower; type of inflorescence.
- Size, colour and shape of flowers and bud.

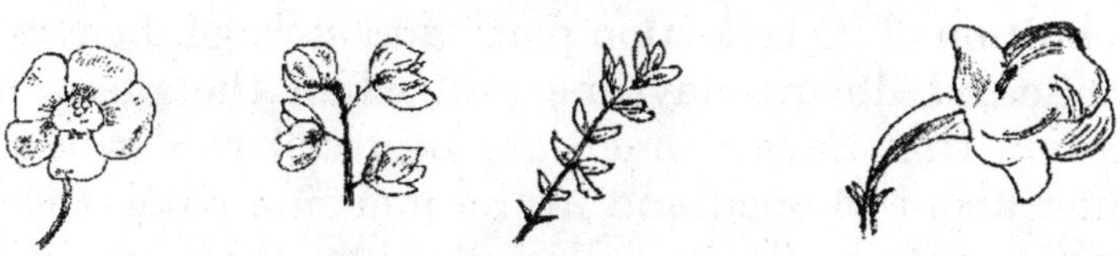

Flowers

Fruits

- Approximate size.
- Shape, colour when young or ripe.
- Seed present or not.
- Size, shape and colour of the seeds.

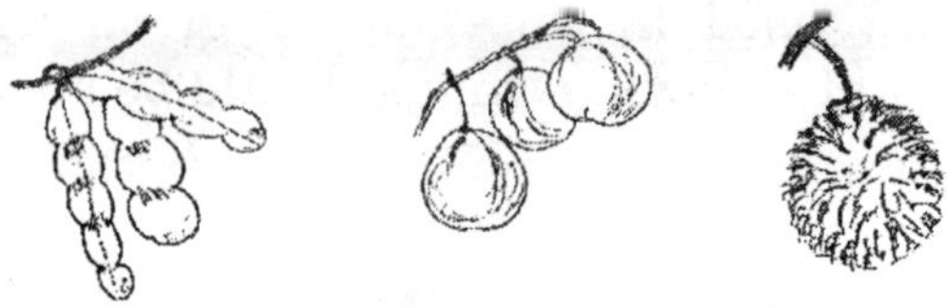

Fruits

Bark

- Present or not.
- Colour and texture (smooth or rough).

During the survey interesting folk uses of ethnoveterinary medicinal plants have come to light which are not mentioned in literature related to medicinal plants. The collected medicinal plants were identified upto species level with the help of floras (Hooker, 1872-1897; Sharma and Tiagi, 1979; Singh and Shetty, 1987-1993; Bhandari, 1990; Almeida, 1998-2004). Final confirmation of the identified plants was done from FRI Herbarium, Dehradun. All the collected specimens were deposited in the Herbarium of Laboratory of Ethnobotany and Agrostology, Department of Botany, College of Science, M.L. Sukhadia University, Udaipur for authentication of information and further references. The information about the medicinal properties of plants is given by mentioning their Botanical name, local name, habitat, part/s used and the mode of their administration.

Collection

Time of collection of plant material is an important thing. The content of the active ingredient may depend on the plant part, stage of growth, season of harvest, method of handling during collection, physical condition of its collection place and storage. Leaves and stems are best collected during daytime and when the plant is about to bloom. Flowers that have a smell are best collected when the flower buds are just about to open and in the morning when the sun is still low. Other flowers should be collected when they are in full bloom. Sometimes, collection should be done in batches since flowers do not bloom at the same time. Unless the remedy says that unripe fruits will be used, fruits should be collected when they are ripe. Fleshy fruits which deteriorate rapidly should be gathered when they are somewhat ripe, preferably in the early morning or at nightfall. Seeds are usually collected from thoroughly ripened fruits. Some dry-textured fruits fall off the plant or split open easily when fully ripened. As a result, seeds are easily scattered and lost. It is advisable to collect such fruits as soon as they start ripening. Barks should be collected when the plants are in bloom or in vigorous growth. Barks should be collected from the trunk and branches. Roots and other underground parts (e.g., rhizome, rootstock, stem tuber, bulb and stolon) are best collected when the plant is in full growth. After collection, sorting and cleaning should be done.

Drying

Air-drying is the best way of drying herbal plants. Drying at high temperature will destroy plant ingredients. Spread the plant materials thinly and evenly over an old newspaper, a bamboo mat, or chicken-wire screen. Put in the shade until the materials are dry. Drying can be done through artificial heat, especially in the rainy season. Heating devices vary from one place to another. After drying cutting, trimming, grinding and chopping should be done

- To increase the efficacy of the plants materials.
- To allow more active ingredients to go into the preparation.
- To reduce the toxicity or adverse effects of certain drugs.
- To shorten the duration of drying.
- To make the plant material more convenient to store.

Storing

Medicinal plants should be properly stored to preserve their quality. Otherwise, they may be attacked by insects, mites and fungus. Storage can also ensure the continuous supply and availability of the materials whenever they are needed. Dried plants should be kept in covered plastic containers or bottles. These should be covered tightly and kept in a cool, dry place away from sunlight. Label the container properly with the name of the plant and the date when it was collected. Do not use any stored herbal plant which has molds or is discolored.

Preparation of herbal veterinary medicine

Plant materials can be either fresh or dry, depending on the need and preparation. If dried plants are to be used as a substitute for fresh parts, adjust the quantity or the weight since water is lost during drying.

Decoction

Boil the plant parts in water, preferably for 15-20 minutes from the time the water has started boiling. Some healers recommend boiling the plant materials until the original volume of the water is reduced to one half. Some plants are soaked or moistened. Ideally, plant materials should be decocted twice in order to extract their active ingredients thoroughly. Strain or filter the liquid either while it is still hot or after cooling.

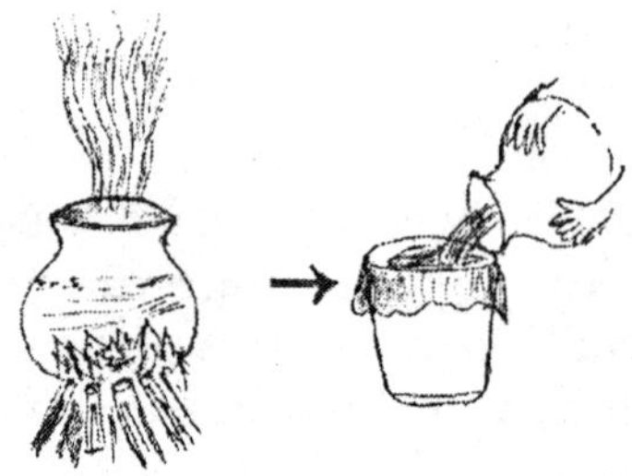

Decoction

Infusion

Pour hot or cold water onto the fresh or dry plant material and allow it to stand. Cover the preparation tightly to stop important ingredients from being lost. The length of time needed to prepare an infusion depends on the type of plant material and whether the water is hot or cold. In general, hot infusions need to stand for only 5-15 minutes; cold infusions may require up to 24 hours. Filter the preparation (and allow hot liquid to cool) before administering to the sick animal.

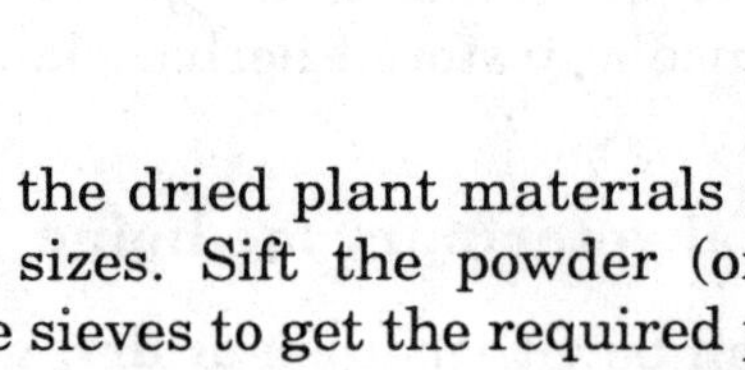

Infusion

Powder

Pound and grind the dried plant materials into coarse, intermediate or fine particle sizes. Sift the powder (once or several times) through coarse or fine sieves to get the required particle size.

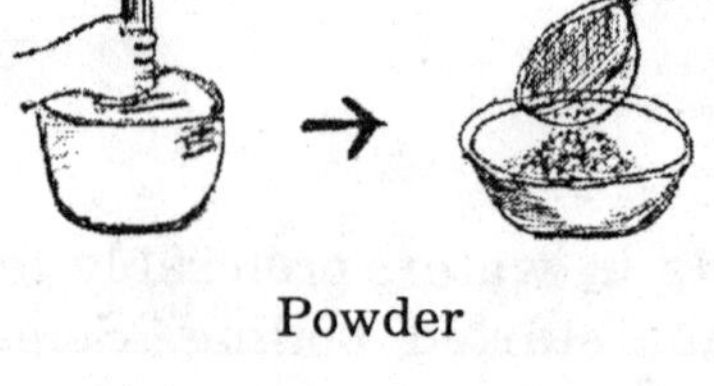

Powder

Juice

Pound the fresh plant materials, then pass them through a cheesecloth or any fine piece of cloth in order to get the juice. Or you may just squeeze the plant parts to extract the juice.

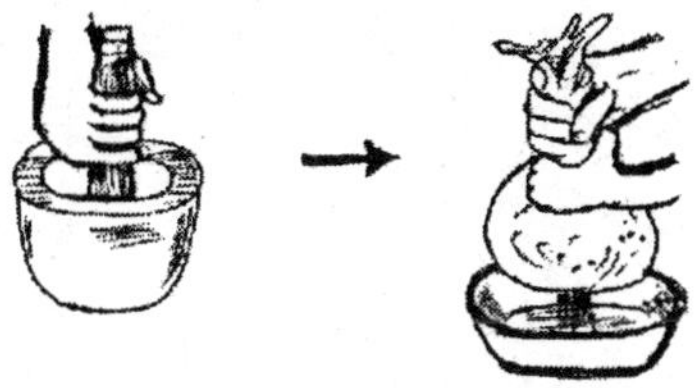

Juice

Poultice or paste

A poultice is a moist, semisolid preparation which is applied directly on the skin. Prepare it by grinding the plant materials (either fresh or dry), sometimes with a little oil, water, molasses, honey, or other liquids.

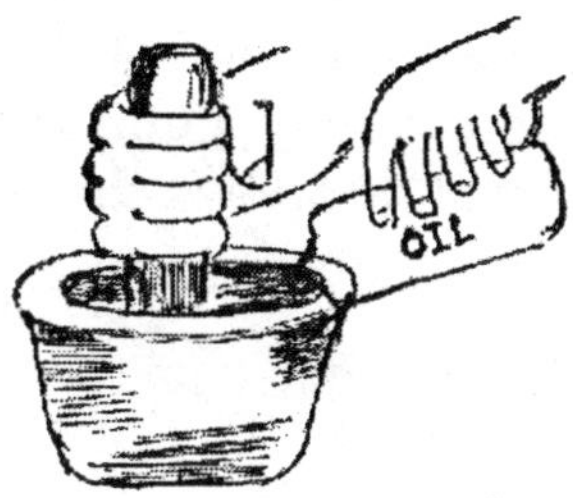

Poultice or paste

Bolus

A bolus is made by pounding fresh or dried plant material' and adding sufficient binding agent such as honey or molasses. Roll it or shape it with your hand to make a round or oval ball

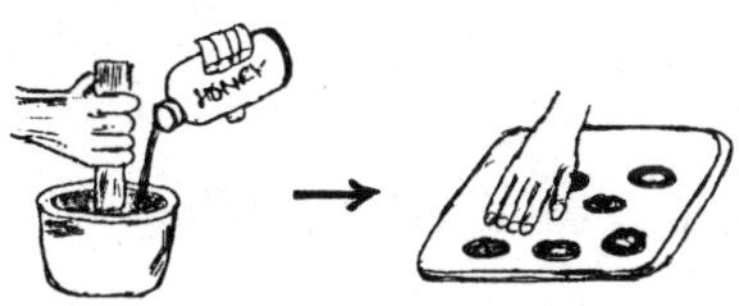

Bolus

Application of herbal medicine

Drenching

The application of liquid preparation through the mouth is called drenching. It can be used for swine, ruminants and poultry. Hold the head level so that the medicine does not go into the lungs. For swine and ruminants, use a bamboo tube, a softdrink bottle, a wine bottle or a bottle gourd. Use a dropper or straw for poultry.

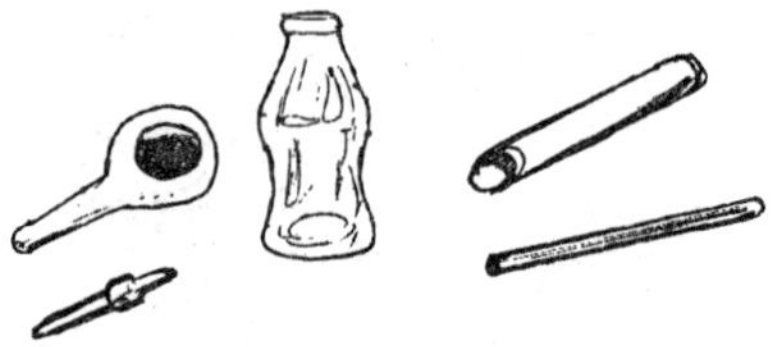

Drenching

Swine

- Tie the animal on its front on the ground and tie it down or ask someone to hold it.
- Tie the snout with a piece of rope. Hold one end of the rope tightly or tie it to a post so the animal's mouth is open and it cannot bite your hands or the bottle. Put the end of the bottle into the mouth and slowly pour the liquid into the mouth. Make sure the animal swallows the liquid.

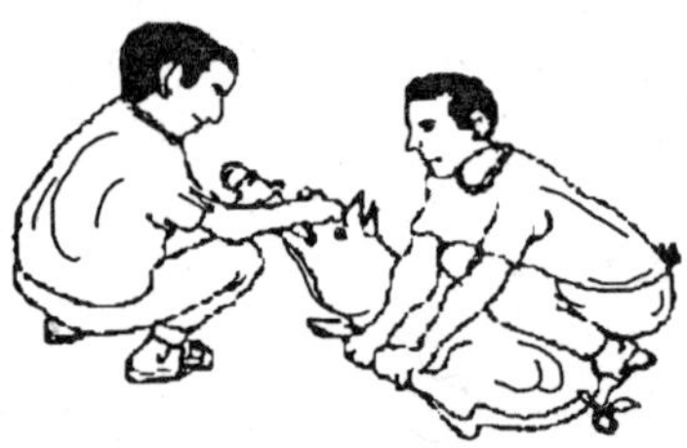

Swine

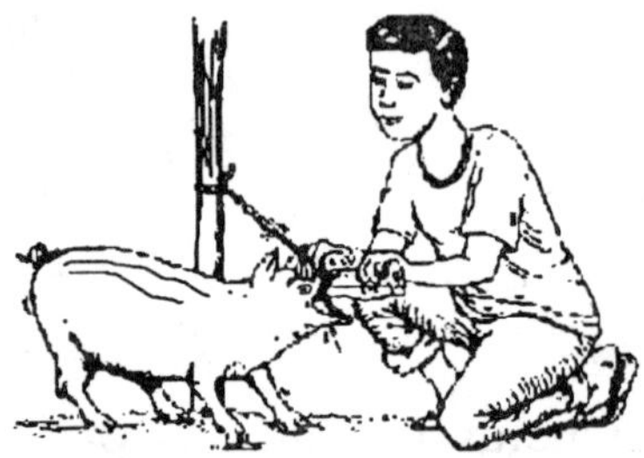

Swine - continue

Ruminants

- Tie the animal to a tree or pole.
- With small ruminants, mount the animal and hold it between your thighs.
- With one hand, hold the upper jaw so that the animal opens its mouth. With cattle and buffaloes, you can use a rope through the nose ring to hold the mouth open. With the other hand, put the end of the bottle in the side of the animal's mouth and slowly pour the liquid into the mouth.

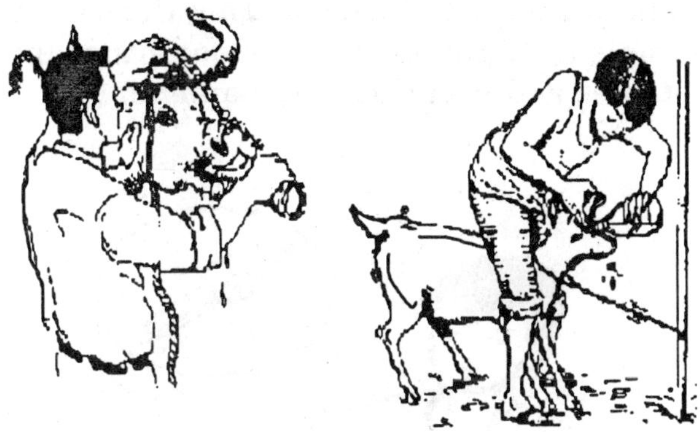

Ruminants

Chickens

Birds can be held by the person who will administer the medicine or by someone else. Use a syringe or dropper or you can use a rice or sorghum straw.

Hold the upper beak with the left thumb or first finger. Push the lower beak down with your finger or the medicine dropper. Hold the head level so the medicine does not go into the lungs.

Drop or squirt the medicine into the mouth.

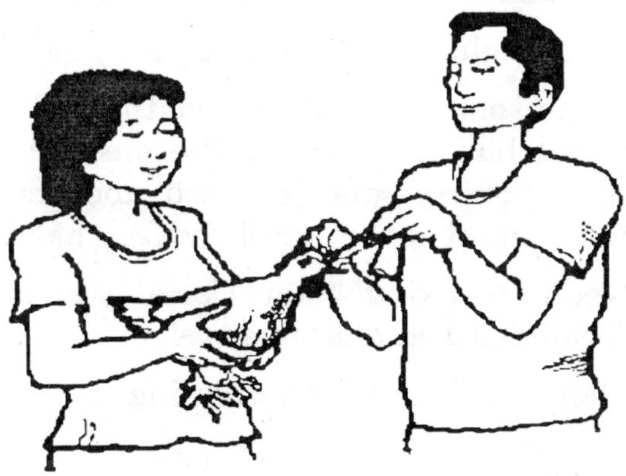

Chickens

Force-feeding

The application of solid preparations through the mouth is called "force feeding". It is used for ruminants, swine and poultry. The procedure is similar to that for drenching. After you have put the solid medicines into the mouth, make sure that the animal swallows them.

In ruminants, this can be done by massaging the throat. An easy way to force-feed animals is to put solid medicines either into a banana or cooked sweet potatoes and feed this to the animal.

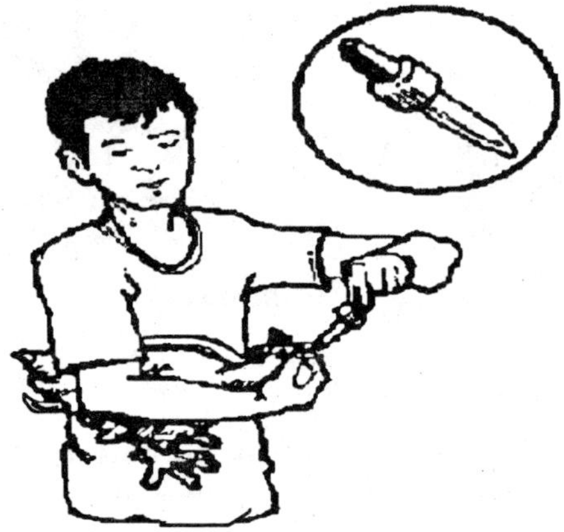

Force-feeding

Medicine mixed with feed and water

- In all species, both liquid and solid medicines can be given with feed and water. They can be:
- Mixed thoroughly with the feed.
- Mixed with some of the feed; give the remaining feed only if the animal has eaten all of the medicated part. To treat individual poultry, put the bird and the medicated feed together under a basket until the feed has been eaten.
- Dissolved in drinking water. Use only as much water as the animal can drink at one time.
- Sprinkled on the feed ("top-dressing").

Topical application

Poultice

- A poultice is a soft, usually heated preparation that is applied to a sore or inflammation.
- If necessary, keep the poultice on if necessary by tying a cloth or strip of banana trunk or coconut leaves over it.
- Poultices are used for swine, ruminants and poultry.

Fomentation

A fomentation is a warm, moist substance (such as a wet cloth) applied to the affected parts of the body. It is used to ease pain and inflammation in swine and ruminants.

Compress

A compress is similar to a fomentation, but is always dry.

This is used for swine and ruminants.

Direct application

Rub the preparation directly on the affected part.

This is used for swine, ruminants and poultry.

Nasal application

Drop medicine directly into the nostril or apply it as vapour as shown in the illustrations. This is used in all species.

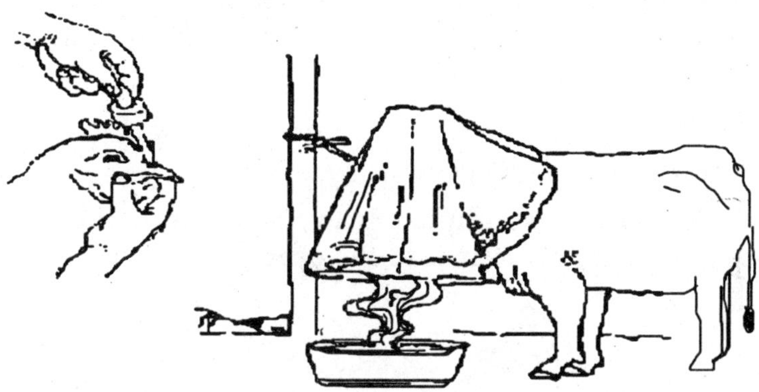

Nasal application

Vaginal application

This application is used in cows that have an infection of the birth canal, for example: after retained placenta or other birth difficulties.

To apply solid medicines

1 Clip the nails, clean hands thoroughly and then apply vegetable oil to them as a lubricant.

2 Clean the animal's vulva with soap and warm water.

3 Take the medicine in one hand and cup this hand into a cone-shape.

4 Insert this hand into the vagina when the muscles of the birth canal are relaxed (for instance, between contractions during birth). Leave the medicine in the vagina and slowly pull your hand out.

To flush the vagina with liquids

1 Clean and wash the stalk of a papaya leaf and lubricate its tip with vegetable oil.

2 Insert the stalk slowly about 10 cm deep into the vagina.

3 Pour the liquid medicine into the vagina through the hollow stalk until the liquid flows over .

Anal application

This can be used for ruminants and swine.

1 Shape the medicine into a small ball.

2 Carefully push it into the animal's anus. If this is difficult, dip the ball into the water or oil before inserting it in the anus.

In the eye

This can be used in all species.

Use a rice straw, sorghum straw, medicine dropper or plastic dropper. Drip remedy directly into the eyes.

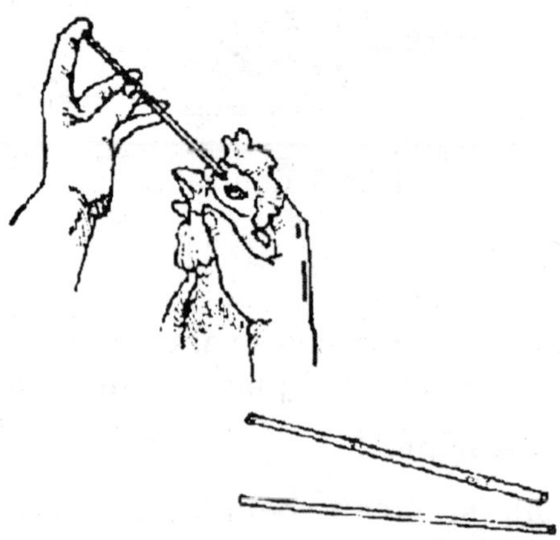

In the eye

Fumigation

- Fumigation is the use of smoke to drive away insects.

- Dried leaves are burned. Now fire is covered with fresh banana leaves to make a lot of smoke.

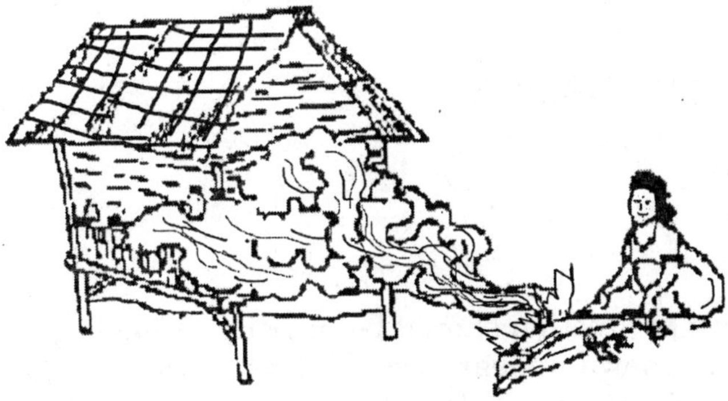

Fumigation

Hanging bouquet

Bind plants into a bouquet and hang inside the houses. This can be used for poultry, swine and ruminants.

Chapter 3

ANIMAL DISEASES

Animal in production should be healthy. A healthy animal is alert and active in general appearance. It is well aware of its surroundings and walks easily with regular steps. The eyes are bright wide open without any discharge at the corners. The nostrils, muzzle and mouth cavity are moist and shining. The skin coat is glossy. The ears are responsive to the sounds. The respiration, dung and urine are normal and without unusual odor. Animal feeds and ruminates regularly and responds to the call of the owner. The tail is in continuous movement to drive away the flies.

Animal Diseases

Predisposing causes of diseases

Adverse climate and weather conditions, *viz* heavy rain, severe cold or severe heat, reduce the natural resistance of the animal body to the diseases. Age of the animal, pollution of water and air, poor feed such as mouldy hay and excessive green crops, excessive work, hereditary conditions etc. are also the pre-disposing causes to the occurrence of diseases.

Disease, in a general sense is deviation from the normal condition of the animal. The animal in health and diseases can be spotted out easily from the signs and animal behaviour. The sick animal looks dull with rough coat, dry external mucous membrane and change in respiration, pulse and temperature. Animal does not feed. It does not respond to the owner and sometimes bites or licks the manger. Urine and dung may alter in smell and consistency. Often animal may lie down and is unable to get up. On the basis of mode and occurrence of diseases these are classified as follows:

Nature of diseases

(i) Acute and chronic diseases: Acute disease starts quickly and runs a short course whereas chronic disease runs for a longer or sometimes indefinite time. Anthrax, haemorrhagic septicemia, etc are acute diseases while Tuberculosis and Johne's diseases are chronic ones.

(ii) Epizootic diseases: Diseases of animals which spread rapidly over a large area (e.g. Rinderpest) are known as epizootic and correspond to the word epidemic, which is used to describe the diseases which spread rapidly amongst human beings.

(iii) Enzootic diseases : This describes a disease which is continuously present in a population of animals, but does not spread rapidly like epizootic.

(iv) Sporadic diseases: This term denotes diseases which appear suddenly from time to time and they are, otherwise, not normally present in an animal population.

(v) Zoonotic diseases : This denotes diseases, which are communicable from animals to human being, some examples are: Brucellosis, Tuberculosis etc.

(vi) Non-infectious and non-contagious diseases: Diseases caused by factors other than living organisms as described above are included in the group of non-infectious diseases. Such diseases may result from a low level of nutrition, lack of vitamins or minerals, hereditary conditions, excessive production of hormones, formation of tumors, mechanical injuries and lesions (cuts, abscesses, ulcers and fractures), poisoning and such other conditions. These diseases are not transmissible from one animal to another. Non-infectious diseases can be classified into following categories:

(1) Common non-Infectious diseases

(2) Production diseases

(3) Deficiency diseases

(4) Common Poisoning.

***(vii) Infectious and contagious diseases*:** Diseases caused by living organism are called infectious diseases. They can spread from one animal to another. Diseases which are transmitted by direct or indirect contact are called contagious. The infectious/contagious diseases are caused by the bacteria, virus, protozoa, parasites and fungi etc.

Non-infectious and non-contagious diseases

(1) Common non-Infectious diseases

In developed countries livestock holders are more particular for prevention of diseases than treatment. They prefer to take measures to keep the animal healthy and resist the disease. They now prefer to use home remedies for animal treatment and call the veterinarian only when it is absolutely necessary. There is also an increasing trend to use harmless, cheap and effective herbal medicines for animal treatment. When the treatment of the sick animal is attempted, the following points may be taken into consideration. In a particular village/area, if many animals are sick at a time with similar symptoms, it may not be a simple disease. It may rather be an infectious disease. Under these circumstances, immediately notify the nearest veterinarian. Before the aid arrives, isolate the sick animals and keep them away from the healthy animals. Do not drag the dead animal on the road. Do not give it to butcher for skinning until the opinion of the veterinarian is obtained. Animal dying of infectious diseases should be buried. Change the pasture. Disinfect the common water troughs. The left over feed and straw/hay of such animal should be burnt. Animals should be vaccinated periodically as scheduled and directed by veterinarian. The precautionary measures and the checks for infectious diseases should be followed correctly in appropriate schedule. The treatment for non infectious diseases with routine remedies should be attempted. Cheap, effective herbal drugs for simple and common conditions can be successfully used by the livestock holders and farmers and disease can be prevented. The animal health care at such a preliminary stage would contribute to increase animal production.

Inflammation : This term is used to denote the reaction of the body to overcome injuries, irritants, fractures and some other disease conditions. In this process, the affected part becomes red, feels hot, swollen and painful and does not function properly. In acute inflammation, if the cause is removed and the part is given rest with hot packs applied over the affected area, the recovery takes place quickly. In chronic inflammation, heat and redness are not very much marked. However, there is slight swelling on the affected part with slight hardness.

Fever : This term indicates a rise in body temperature which is usually accompanied by loss of appetite, increase respiration and pulse, sweating and shivering and decreased urination. Fever can be due to sudden change in weather, viral, bacterial or protozoal diseases and due to sun stroke. A simple method to feel fever is holding the base of the ear.

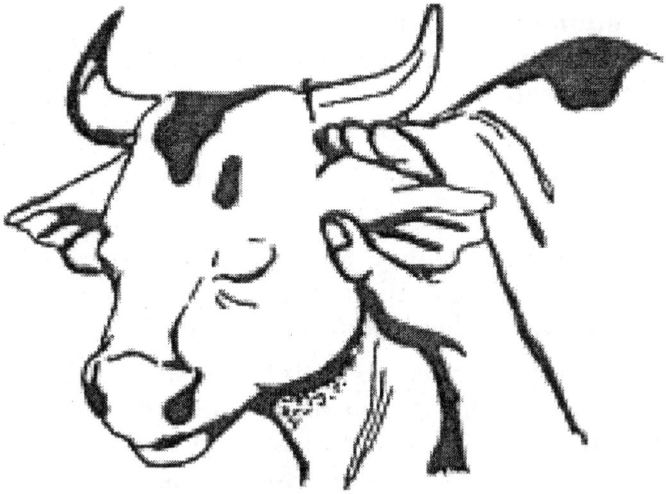

Fractures : Any kind of crack or break usually due to accidents or severe injury to the bony tissue is referred as fracture. Painful swelling of the affected part is the earliest sign exhibited by the animal. Fracture of the limb is manifested by severe lameness and presence of crackling sound on palpation.

Skin diseases: Skin is the mirror of animal health. It performs specific functions for keeping animal healthy. Skin helps to maintain the normal body temperature, control the body fluids and electrolytes balance, synthesizes vitamin D with the help of sunlight, protects the body from bacterial invasions, etc. Moreover animal skin is valuable for its hide. Hide from the healthy skin fetches more value. Production of wool and mohair from healthy skin of sheep and goat is more valuable. Thus the care of the skin plays an important role in animal industry. Heat, cold, moisture, physical and chemical substances, bacteria, virus, fungus, parasites, mineral deficiencies, skin injuries, accidents, allergic conditions, etc. play a considerable role in skin diseases.

Wounds: Bleeding occurs from wound. The cut skin separates and the part is painful. If the wound is not treated, flies attack the wound and maggots are formed. On farms, the wounds are caused by sharp agricultural implements with signs of bleeding, rendering animal unable to walk.

Bruised wounds : Superficial wounds develop if the animal rubs the skin on rough surfaces. They are very painful.

Lacerated wounds : When the animal is bruised with barbed wire and sharp objects accidentally, it develops such wound causing irregular skin cuts.

Punctured wounds : Penetration of sharp instruments cause deep punctured wounds. In such wounds, deep bacterial infections lead to tetanus or sepsis.

Incised wounds : While performing surgery, the wound is created by cutting with knife. These wounds are with regular skin contour.

Crushed wounds: Injury on the skin with non sharp objects causes crushed wounds (contusion). Such wounds may show internal bleeding. If unattended they end in gangrene.

Abscess : It is a rounded hot painful swelling full of pus. It occurs due to injury from irritant on the skin or infected wound or as a result of internal disease. It may be caused due to infected/contaminated instruments, syringe and needles. It can be prevented by keeping animals clean and well fed, using sterilized instrument, syringe and needles and proper dressing of the open wounds.

Burns : There are some disease conditions which involve only topical applications and can be attended by the farmers. The animals exposed to lightening with involvement of large body area can be treated with potato mash if nothing is available.

Hoof wounds, warts, and tumors: Hoof wounds, warts and tumors on the hoof and in between the hooves are removed with knife and treated with dry powder of alum, ferrous sulphate and copper sulphate in equal proportion for two days followed by wound healing powder.

Antifungal: Ringworm, eczema etc. are fungal diseases commonly seen in animals.

External parasitic diseases: External parasites such as lice, ticks, fleas, mosquitoes etc. are inimical to animal production.

Diseases of digestive system

Diseases of the digestive system can be divided into three groups for approach from the farmer's point of view. (i) Routine general complaints which are the symptoms of some specific diseases. (ii) Infectious diseases. (iii) Worms.

Ulcers in mouth cavity

Ulcers may develop in the oral mucus membrane, tongue, gums, cheeks and lips. Ulcers are also symptom of infectious disease like foot and mouth diseases, rinderpest, etc. It may develop due to injury, eating irritant substances and constipation etc. Due to ulcer mouth smell and salivation increases. Animal can not chew properly and food drops down from mouth.

Off feed/ Anorexia: Anorexia is a sign of the disease. Anorectic animal refuses to take food. This also happens after the animal over eats. The animal goes to dustbins and licks earth and gobbles waste and rotten food. Over and under worked animals also become off feed.

Impaction of rumen

Intake of non succulant dry feeds, restricted watering, accidental over eating of grains, especially in harvesting season, are main causes of impaction. Impaction is also a sign of some more serious infectious or non-infectious diseases. Animal is indisposed after about 12 hours of over eating. Kicks the belly with hind legs. Gets up and sits down. The left flank feels solid on pressure with hand. Rumination stops. Dung becomes thick and dry or stops or sometimes ends in smelling diarrhoea. Respiration and pulse rate increase, sometimes temperature also increases. Animal lies down and may die in 48 to 72 hours.

Constipation

Constipation occurs in diseases of stomach and intestine. Animal habituated to eat clay, plastic waste and non-digestible food gets constipated. Decreased water intake also leads to constipation. Animal exhibits signs of dullness, rough coat, poor rumination and off feed. Dung is dry and scanty or even stops passing.

Flatulence: Gas is normally formed in the rumen from the fermentation of feed and is belched out through the gullet. Bloat or tympany occurs when gas accumulates in rumen and animal cannot get rid of it without help. When gas is mixed with food it forms froth and cause frothy bloat.

Occurrence of bloat is based on type of feed and the amount of water given to the animal. Sudden change to certain type of feed ration also causes bloat. When animal consumes excessive quantity of tender succulent leguminous, excessive nitrogenous fodder or less fibrous feeds, bloat occurs. Cabbage leaves, feeds sprinkled with urea are also associated with bloat. Sprouted or unwanted tender plants of sorghum, water soaked bean *(Dolichos lablab)* and plants containing hydrocyanic acid and glycosides cause severe bloat. Other causes of bloat are, blockage of food pipe, constipation causing plants or foreign matter, paralysis of nerve and infections.

Acute (severe) bloat suddenly occurs, after grazing lush green fodder or after over feeding with fermentative feeds. Left flank region gets distended. Animal is in pain and distress and stops drooling, breathing is rapid. animal stops eating or chewing and kicks with hind legs. Muzzle becomes cold. Chronic bloat occurs very often and comparatively less distention of left flank is noticed in it.

Colic

Conditions like impaction, bloat and indigestion lead to colic. The animal is restless. Sits down and gets up frequently. It looks and kicks at the abdomen.

Internal injury to stomach

Animals some time swallow nails, pieces of wire, needles etc. Through the second stomach (Reticulum), they pierce the diaphragm and reach the chest cavity and injure the heart. Many a times these pieces lodged in the pericardium of the heart which is characterized by swelling on the left side near the heart, and may form a big abscess. Animal becomes off feed and goes on wasting. Production is decreased. Skin coat appears dry and rough. Body temperature may increase. There is straining at defecation and urination. In such conditions, take the advice of veterinary surgeon at the earliest. Surgery is required to be performed for removing such objects.

Diarrhoea

Calves get diarrhoea often. It may be due to bacteria or indigestion. Adult animals get diarhoea after grazing on pastures or due to irritants. Defecation is more frequent than normal. Diarrhoea may be watery, green, yellow, mixed with mucus and smelling, mucus and some times pus is noticed in diarrhoea. Hind quarters are soiled. Animal becomes dull with sunken eyes, weak and dehydrated

Diseases of Respiratory and Circulatory system

Respiratory systems

Cold and cough

This is a sign of some systemic or upper respiratory tract diseases. Sudden changes in the weather, over-crowding of animals, moist condition in animal houses, exposure to cold, wetting in rain, infection due to bacteria, virus, fungus, parasites and allergy are some of the causes of cold and cough. Animal is dull and off feed. There is coughing, sneezing and eye and nasal discharge. Body temperature may rise, animal tries to rub the nose with tree or wall with difficulty in breathing.

Pneumonia

Cold, coryza, sudden change in weather and fever are some of the predisposing causes of pneumonia. Bacteria, virus and parasites attack the lung and the wind pipe to set up the disease. Drenching pneumonia commonly occurs when there is accidental entry of the drenching liquid into the windpipe. Animal becomes dull and off feed. There is difficulty in breathing. Body temperature increases. Nasal discharge and cough may be seen. Animal may keep the head hanging down.

Diseases of Urinary System: Inflammation of kidney (nephritis), urinary bladder and ureters and stoppage of urine due to calculi in the kidneys or urethra are some of the common manifestations of diseases of urinary system. In all these diseases there may be bacterial infection or injury to the affected part because of crystal formation. In urinary calculi especially in bullock, there is concentration of mineral salts and colloids in urinary tract causing inflammation of kidney, ureters, bladder or urethra.

In urinary disease the most common symptom is urinary colic; here the urine becomes scanty and stops when calculi obstructs the passage. Animal kicks, strains, and becomes restless. It tries to strain often for urination. If the animal is tied on dry place, wetting of soil due to urine is not seen. On complete stoppage of urine animal goes untruly, runs amok, salivates, feeding and rumination stops. After two to three days, the urinary blader ruptures and these symptoms subside. Animal sits down. There is smell from the mouth, skin coat becomes rough and temperature may rise.

Diseases of reproductive system

Reproductive system plays a vital role in animal production and effective animal husbandry development programme. Some commonly occurring disease conditions requiring first aid treatment by farmers / livestock owners are as follows:

Swelling (inflammation) of Penis

Penis gets swollen, due to some infection or by crushing due to weight on sitting on hard surfaces or by injury. Wounds, injury or faulty matting, etc. can also cause swelling of penis. Penis does not protrude properly and urination becomes painful. Blood may be seen in urine. Animal licks the affected part, becomes restless and wound and ulcer may develop subsequently.

Inflammation of uterus **(Metritis):** It may be acute or chronic, normally occurs after parturition. Infection during parturition, retention of placenta, abortion and removal of calf by hand under unhygienic conditions may lead to metritis. Temperature may increase in acute metritis. Foul smelling vaginal discharge associated with pus and blood is common. Milk production decreases and the animal is off feed with cessation of rumination.

Prolapse of uterus

In this condition uterus or vagina protrudes out through the vulva. This condition may occur due to excessive straining before or after parturition. It may also be associated with some diseases of the uterus or due to accumulation of urine in the bladder. Animals having gone through many parturitions are more prone to this condition. The uterus protrudes and hangs out side the vulva. In partial prolapse, the uterine mass is seen protruding out when the animal is sitting. If left untreated, the exposed part gets injured and infected, causing development of wounds and ulcers. Birds prick on the exposed part and cause injury. Animal continue to strain with a rise in body temperature. Milk production drops or stops.

Retained placenta

In normal parturition the placenta is expelled in 3-6 hours. If this does not happen then it requires manual removal. Difficult parturition, atony of uterine muscles, improper feeding, infections and inflammation of uterus are some of the reasons for retained placenta.

Abortion: Sometimes the animal throws out the developing foetus from the uterus. This is called abortion. This may normally happen after five or six months of pregnancy or in advance pregnancy Abortion may occur due to many reasons like, imbalanced feed, deficiency of vitamins, following drenching of strong purgatives or abortifacient drugs, accidental falls, feeding of fungus infected grains and unripe sorghum or infectious diseases. Aborted animals should be treated as if they have normally been parturated.

Sore teats and teat wounds

A common condition in milking cattle is a sore teat with cracking of the skin usually caused by "wet milking." It may also result from cow pox and foot and mouth disease. The condition starts as small swellings in the skin of the teats or udder which become blisters and then turn into small abscesses containing pus. Wounds of teats are often caused by cuts and injuries from barbed wire and thorny bushes. Wound of this kind can lead to mastitis or inflammation of the udder.

(2 & 3) Production and deficiency Diseases

Amongst farm animals, mostly dairy cows and pregnant ewes suffer from production diseases. The incidence of production diseases is highest in high milk producing animals and occurs immediately after parturition and in early lactation. During this period there is high turnover of fluids, solids and soluble organic materials. Any sudden variation in intake, secretion and excretion leads to alterations in the internal environment of the animal. This makes animal prone to suffer from characteristic metabolic diseases. The major factors leading to metabolic diseases are nutritional deficiency, production stress, management practices, and environmental variations. There are large number of deficiency diseases, prominent being Avitanimosis-A, copper, cobalt and zinc deficiencies. Calcium and phosphorous deficiency also lead to various disorders. Proper feeding regimen and supplement feeding of mineral mixture will avert major deficiency diseases. Because of their high incidence and production importance, important metabolic diseases are briefed here.

Milk fever

This disease is also known as parturient paresis. Heavy milkers suffer from this disease most commonly. The disease may occur in late pregnancy or 2-10 days after parturition and is characterized by hypocalcaemia, general muscular weakness, circulatory collapse and loss of consciousness. Mostly occurs within 48 hours after parturition.

Heavy milkers pass more calcium in colostrum and milk. Serum calcium deficiency eventually occurs which leads to milk fever. Deficiency of magnesium is also a contributory factor. Insufficiency of parathyroid gland which controls calcium secretion and its mobilization is also responsible for milk fever.

This disease is rare in second lactation and occurs more frequently in animals in 3rd to 5th lactation. Initially there is excitement and tetany with hypersensitiveness and muscle tremor. There may be shaking of head, protrusion of tongue and animal does not move or reluctant to move. Animal becomes recumbent, looks drowsy, unable to rise, muzzle becomes dry, skin and extremities feel cool, body temperature goes subnormal, eyes are dry, pupil dilated, weak pulse with increased rate and ruminal stasis with constipation are observed. In advanced stage there is lateral recumbery with flaccidity, increased heart rate and inpalpable pulse, bloat, coma and death.

Ketosis

This disease is also known as acetonaemia, ketonaemia, ketonuria, hypoglycaemia. Heavy milking animals can get this disease usually 15-20 days after parturition. It also occur in winter season in housed animals. A secondary ketosis may also develop due to loss of appetite as a result of abomasal displacement, traumatic reticulitis, metritis and mastitis.

Ketone bodies increase due to defective metabolism of carbohydrate. Excessive or very less feeding of imbalanced feed having more nitrogen and less carbohydrate will cause carbohydrate deficiency. In such a condition, to maintain body function, animal draws energy from body fat, which results in increase of ketone bodies and acetone in blood, causing the disease. Feeding more concentrates and less dry roughages also contributes to the disease.

Ketosis can occur early after parturition or rarely may be seen up to 60 days. Milk production and feed intake decreases. Animal stands with drooling head with closed eyes. Dung may be hard or soft like diarrhoea. Tympany may occur. Ketonic odour comes in breath and often in milk. Sometimes the animal gets excited and moves in circles. Salivation, licking, chewing, tremors and tetany may be seen. Body temperature may also increase.

Lactation tetany (Hypomagnesaemic tetany, grass tetany, grass stagger)

It is a fatal disease occurring in lactating cows, characterized by hypomagnesemia and hypocalcaemia and clinically by tonic and clonic muscular spasms and convulsions. It is most common in first two months after calving.

Grazing pasture deficient in magnesium and pasture top dressed with nitrogen and potash rich fertilizer and stress of lactation are predisposing factors for grass tetany. Unusually alert, hyperesthesia, incoordination, staggering gait condition, temperature rises after severe muscle exertion, the pulse and respiratory rates are high and the animal dies even before the treatment is given. In subacute cases inappetence, exaggerated movements, urination, defecation, decreased milk production and ruminal stasis are observed and animal may recover spontaneously.

(4) Common poisoning

Poisoning in animals occur due to consumption of some plants or due to accidental access to poisoning material. The common poisoning in animals is as follows:

(1) Sorghum (Jowar) poisoning or hydrocyanic acid poisoning. This poisoning occurs when animals graze on unripe sorghum. This poisoning is also seeing when animals consume non watered sorghum oat etc.

(2) Nitrate/Nitrite poisoning due to feeding/grazing nitrogenous plants.

(3) Pesticide/insecticide poisoning due to consumption of plants contaminated with Pesticides/insecticides.

(4) Lead poisoning due to consumption of fodder contaminated with lead or due to drinking contaminated water.

(5) Fluorosis: It occurs due to feed and water contamination with fluoride. For treatment of the poisoning cases, immediate assistance of veterinarian should be sought.

If source of poisoning is known, immediately discontinue the source. Feeding eggs, charcoal and milk and purging are the steps to be followed at first hand. However expert's intervention is necessary.

(VI) Infectious Diseases

1. Bacterial diseases

***Anthrax** : It is fatal disease characterized by high temperature, bleeding from natural orifice, reduced lactation, abortion and some times sudden death also occur.

Black quarter: It is characterized by sudden death, high temperature, lameness, reduced lactation, swelling on hind quarters, shoulder region. Crepitating sound on pressure.

***Brucellosis:** It is a sexual disease characterized by abortions in late pregnancy in female, sterility in male, retention of placenta, metritis and swelling of testicles

Calf dyptheria: In caves this disease is characterized by fever, necrotic stomatitis (ulcers in the mouth cavity), salivation, acute toxemia and nasal discharge

Calf paratyphoid: In caves this disease is characterized by anorexia, dullness, high fever, dysentry with tenesmus, putrid smell of faeces, dehydration and emaciation.

White scoure (Enteric collibacillosis): Young calves up to 2-3 weeks are affected by this disease, which is characterized by progressive diarrhoea, emaciation, dehydration, sucken eyes, hind quarters, soiled with fluid feces and sometimes death occurs.

Calf dysentery: This disease is characterized by watery diarrhoea progressive dehydrations and weakness.

Foot Rot: Foot rot or foul in foot is a common problem of cattle, sheep and goats. It is usually caused by bacteria or fungus. Moist ground predisposes the condition. The disease is most commonly seen during autumn and winter. Animals with foot rot goes lame with swelling of the hoof and is unable to bear weight on infected foot. In severe cases, there may be rise of temp, pulse and respiration. The animal may go off feed and rumination gets sluggish. Examination of hoof reveals presence of pus, foul smelling odour and dead tissue in the interdigital space. Foot lesion with vesicles are seen in F.M.D but can be differentiated by absence of mouth lesions in foot rot.

Hemorrhagic septicaemia : In this disease cattle suffer from sudden on set of fever, profuse salivation hot painful swelling under neck region, dewlap and brisket.

Jhone's disease: This disease is common in 2-6 yrs. age group cattle, characterized by long course for several months of emaciation, sub mandibular oedema, diarrhea, dehydration and thirst.

Tetanus: This disease is characterized by Muscle stiffness, profuse sweating, restriction of jaw movements, prolapse of 3rd eye lid, unsteady straddling gait drooling of saliva dilatation of nostrils and fever in late stage.

Tuberculosis : This disease is characterized by emaciation, enlarged lymph nodes, loss of weight, diarrhoea, coughing, bloat, mastitis, metritis and some times death occurs after prolonged illness

Vibriosis (Campylobactor): In this disease cattle suffers from fever, mucoid diarrhea and sporadic dysentery. This disease also causes infertility among cattle.

Wooden tongue (Actinobacillosis): Sudden onset of disease characterized by excessive salivation, swollen and hard tongue, nodules and ulcers on togue, pus with yellowish granule and lymph node enlargement which makes the cattle unable to eat.

Lumpy Jaw (Actinomycosis): This disease is characterized by painless bony swelling of jaws which makes them hard, immovable and causes difficulty in mastication. Dyspnoea, weakness and emaciation also occurs.

Mastitis

It is generally caused by the in production of bacteria into the udder, through the teat orifice and teat canal, Bacteria, also gain entry through cuts, bruises, tears, etc. The usual predisposing cause of mastitis is bad milking practice such as wet milking, lack of cleanliness, rough milking and incomplete striping of teats. Mastitis may spread throughout the herd if precautions are not taken.

In mastitis udder become swollen with diminished milk yield and teats hot and painful. In some cases cows go off feed, does not permit milking, have temperature, loose condition and even die. Early mastitis is generally found if a "stripcup" method of detection is in regular use and the first few drops of milk are smeared onto it. This will show the clots and flakes in positive cases. Chronic mastitis may show few signs of the condition. In such cases, however, the milk may be watery or bloody in appearance, has a bitter taste and lumps or clots may be seen in the first few drops of milk taken from an infected quarter.

2. Viral diseases

Foot and mouth Disease: This disease is characterized by high fever, painful stomatitis, ropy saliva and large vesicles in mouth cavity.

Goat Plague (PPR): Sheep and goat usually suffer from this disease which is characterized by fever, off feed, necrotic ulcer in mouth, discharge from eye and nose and respiration distress.

C.C.P.P. (Contagious Caprine pleuro pneumonia): It is a fatal disease commonly occurs in goats characterized by high temperature, difficult breathing, nasal discharge and higher coughing.

Pneumonia: This disease is characterized by high fever, laboured breathing, blood tinged nasal discharge, weakness and animal appears dull and depressed.

Malignant catarrhal fever: This disease is characterized by erosius stomatitis (ulcers in mouth cavity), high fever, severe dejection, conjunctivitis, haematuria, enlarged lymph nodes, diarrhea and lesions on skin.

Mucosal disease : This disease is characterized by ulcers in the mouth cavity, stomatitis, moderate fever, profuse diarrhoea, dehydration, emaciation, intermittent bloat

Sheep pox & Goat pox : Sheep and goat usually suffer from this disease which is characterized by fever, ulcers in mouth, scabs on hairless parts, Nasal discharge, lacrimation and animal looks dull and depressed.

Blue Tongue: Usually this disease occurs in buffaloes, sheep and goats, which is characterized by fever, dullness, panting, ulcers in mouth, dental pads, swollen face, cyanotic (blue) tongue and lameness.

Rinderpest: This disease is characterized by ulcers in the mouth cavity, stomatitis blood stained saliva, high fever and severe diarrhoea.

Dengue Fever (Three days sickness): This disease is characterized by anorexia, enlargement of peripheral lymph nodes, muscular shivering, sharp fall in milk and eye discharge.

Cowpox and buffalopox: Disease characterized by pox lesions on teat and udder, vesicles formation followed by pustules and scab.

I.B. R./I.P.V. (Infectious Bovine Rhinotracheit / Infectious Pustalar Vulvo-Vaginitis): This disease is characterized by anorexia, fever, nasal discharge difficult breathing, ulcers in mouth, enteritis. pustules on vulva-vagina, conjunctivitis and salivation. Some time abortion also occurs in pregnant animal.

B.V.D (Bovine Viral Diarrhoea): This disease is characterized by anorexia, temperature, ulcers in mouth, lameness, watery diarrhea, dehydration, abortion, ataxia in calves.

Contagious ecthyma : Disease commonly occur in goats and sheep, which is characterized by pustular lesions on muzle and lips. In lambs and kids pneumonia and gastritis occur with fever and high mortality.

Rabies: Due to this disease animals become violent and frenzy. Death occurs in infected animals within 10-15 days.

Protozoa

i. Tick borne (Anaplasmosis): This disease is characterized by fluctuating fever, anorexia, anemia, emaciation, yellow coloured mucous membrane and jaundice.

Babesiosis: This disease is characterized by sudden onset of high fever, anorexia, depression, cessation of rumination, anaemia and sometimes jaundice also occurs.

Theileriosis: This disease is characterized by anorexia, depression and swelling around scrotal area.

ii. Fly borne

Trypanosomiasis (Surra): This is a sexual disease characterized by odema around penis, scrotum and prepuce in males and vulva swollen inguinal lymph nodes, mucopurulent, urethral discharge in females. Cutaneous patches, stiffness of limbs, emaciation, and sometimes fever also occurs.

Internal parasite

Coccidiosis: This disease is characterized by sudden onset of severe diarrhoea, blood stained faeces with foul odour, rectal prolapse, dehydration, anaemia, anorexia and reduced lactation.

Flukes: This disease usually spread in summer and autumn. Due to this disease animal becomes dull, weak, facing poor appetite. In chronic condition animal becomes anaemic, and sometimes death also occurs.

Helminths

Roundworms: This disease is characterized by anorexia, depression, pot belly appearance of abdomen, emaciation, anaemia retarded growth, diarrhea and dermatitis

Tape worms: This disease is characterized by anaemia unthriftness, poor condition of coat, digestive disturbances, constipation and diarrhea.

Trichomoniasis: Sexual disease characterized by infertility, repeat breeding, and abortion.

Round-worms, tape worms and flukes are the common parasites harbouring the digestive tract of animals. When the worm burden increases, the animal gets thin, pale, anemic and dull. There is loss of appetite, diarrhoea, enlarged abdomen, decreased production and death in heavy infestation. Young and poorly nourished animals are more susceptible and problem of parasite is more common in rainy season. Most commonly, animals acquire parasitic infestation after ingestion of food or water contaminated with larvae or eggs.

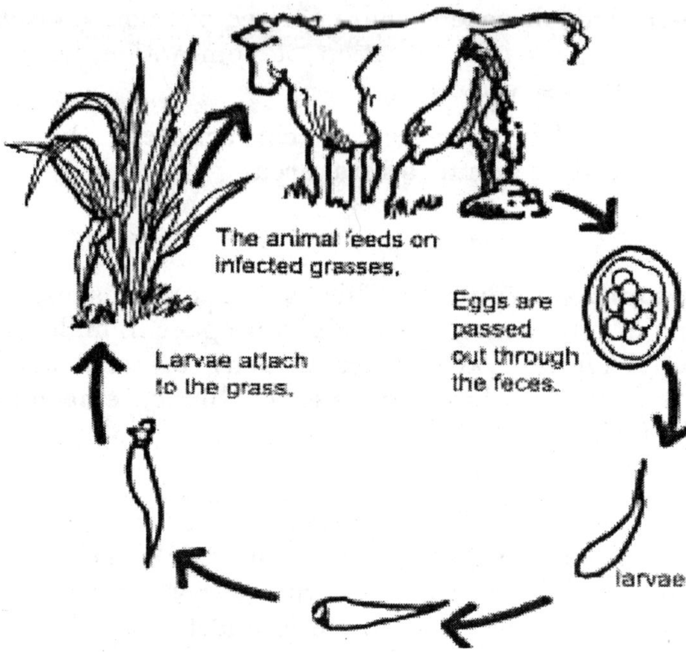

Life cycle of the intestinal worms

External Parasites

Mange, Mite, Ticks and Fly: This disease is characterized by nodules, pustules on the skin, reddening of the skin, scratching, biting, weakness, uneasiness and loss of hairs.

CHAPTER 4

ETHNOVETERINARY REMEDIES : PLANTS

During the ethnoveterinary survey of the study area, folk uses of about 265 ethnoveterinary herbs have been documented. In the following account, plants are arranged alphabetically by botanical names followed by their families in paranthesis, local name in itallics, brief botanical description, ecology, flowering and fruiting and mode of administration.

ENUMERATION

***Abrus precatorius* Linn. (Fabaceae)** *Chirmi, Ratti, Charmoli, Chanboi* (Plate 2)

Copiously branched climber with slender branches; leaves alternate, pinnately compound with numerous deciduous leaflets; flowers small in dense raceme on axillary peduncles or short branches; pods 3 to 5 seeded; seeds red with black blotch around the hilum. Frequent on the hilly tracts in dense forests. Fl. & Fr.: August – January.

Paste of two to three soaked seeds is given to the animals to treat constipation and expelling of retained placenta. Powder of two to three seeds is given to animal with bread for two to four times a day for oestrus induction. Paste of root is applied over mammary glands of animals to treat mastitis. Leaf paste is mixed with starch of rice and given orally to treat anthrax. Leaves are grinded with milk of goat and given orally to treat insect bite.

***Abutilon indicum* (Linn.) Sweet (Malvaceae)** *Kanghi, Jhumka* (Plate 2)

Shrub; leaves simple, petiolate, cordate, nearly entire or irregularly toothed, surface rough with closely felted white hairs, stipules deflexed; flowers axillary pedunculate; fruits of ripe carpels separating from the axis.Common in wastelands, gardens and neglected corners of the cultivated fields. Fl. & Fr.: August - December.

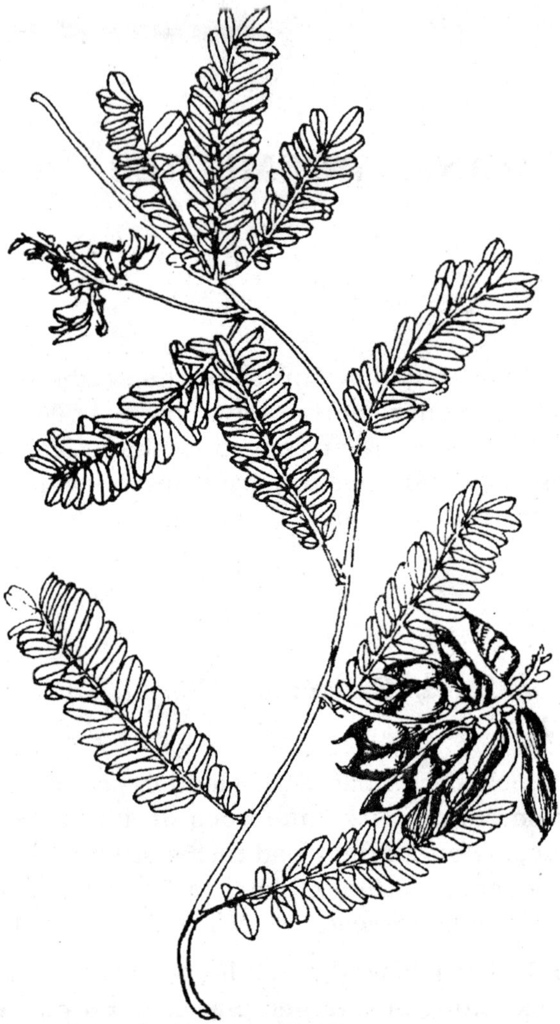

Fig. 1. *Abrus precatorius* Linn.

Paste of about 20 gm seeds is given orally once in a day for relief from constipation. About 500 g leaves are given to the animal along with fodder to treat haematuria. Leaves are grinded with milk and given orally to treat dysentery.

Acacia catechu (L.f.) Willd. (Mimosaceae) *Katha, Khair*

Tree, up to 10 m in height; bark dark greyish brown, 2.25 cm thick; spikes axillary, cylindrical; flowers small, sessile, pale creamy white; fruits flat, pods brown, spiny with a triangular beak at the apex and narrowed at the base; seeds 3-10 per pod. Grow in abundance in drier region. Fl. & Fr: May- September.

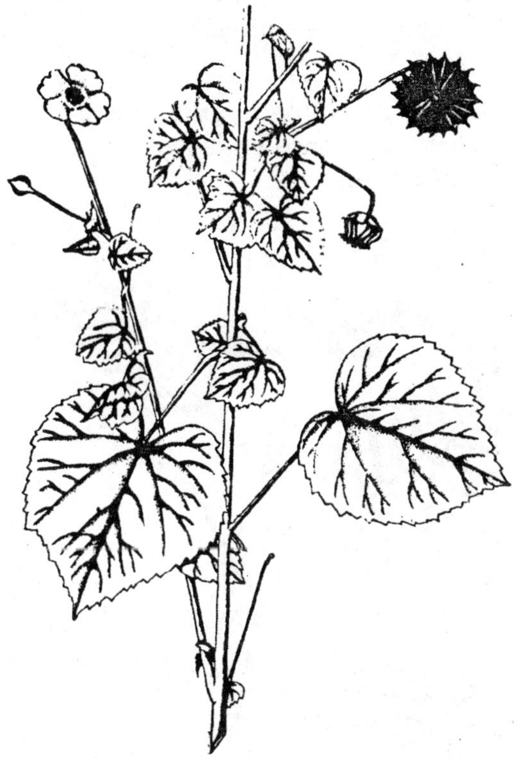

Fig. 2. *Abutilon indicum* (Linn.)

Young leaves and flowers are fed to the animal to induce labour pain.

***Acacia concinna* (Willd.) DC. (Mimosaceae)** *Sikakai, Kochi*

A common, prickly, scandent shrub; leaves bipinnate; flowers in yellow, globose, auxillary heads; pods brown, wrinkled and notched when dry; seeds 6-10 in a pod. Occur in tropical forest throughout India. Fl. & Fr.: May – October.

Seeds are crushed with buttermilk and given orally to treat food poisoning.

***Acacia leucophloea* (Roxb.) Willd. (Mimosaceae)** *Khar, Safed-kikar, Rijua*

Deciduous tree; leaves alternate, compound, stipules spiny; heads yellow, small, not more then 0.62 cm in diameter, flowers small; pods sessile, 10-12 cm in length, sub indehiscent, clothed with pale brown or grey persistent tomentum. Grows in arid, desertic and semi-desertic areas with typical xerophytic characters. Fl. & Fr.: August-February.

Decoction of about 50g roots is given once in a day for 8 days for the treatment of fractured bone. Pods are given to animals along with fodder for oestrus induction.

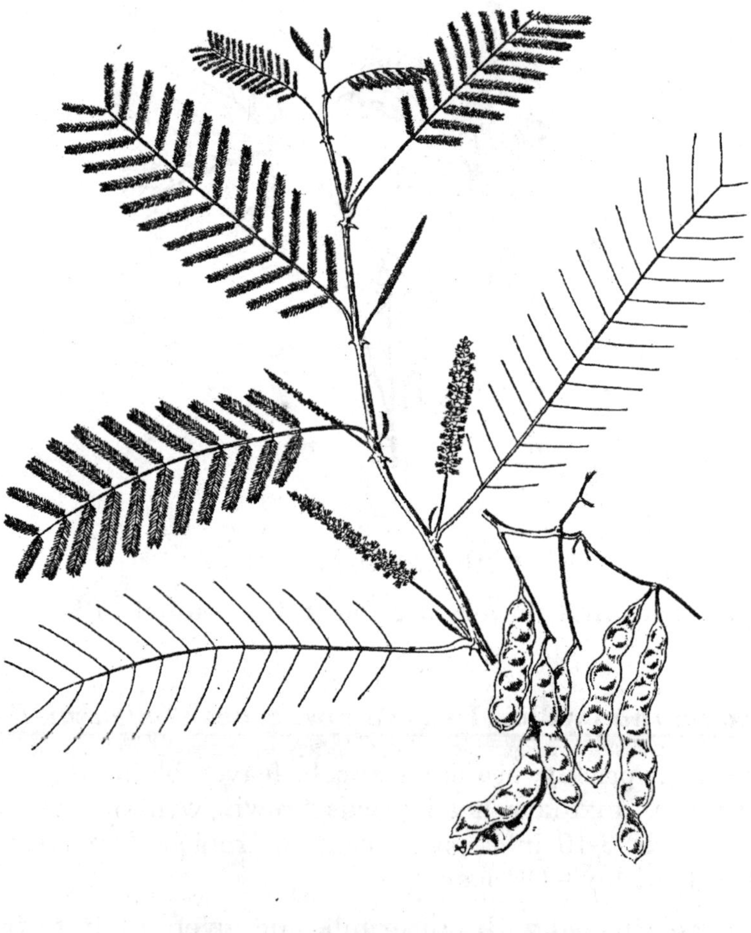

Fig. 3. *Acacia catechu* (L.f.) Willd.

***Acacia nilotica* (Linn.) Willd. ex Del. (Mimosaceae)** *Kikar, Babul, Desi-babul, Babool*

Tree, branchlets straight, finely grey downy; leaves bipinnate, leaf rachis downy with several glands; peduncle short, densely grey downy, profusely bracteate; heads yellow; pods rigid coriaceous, subindehiscent, densely persistently grey-downy, 8 to 12 seeded. Xerophyte, growing scatteredly in crop fields in the drier region of Rajasthan and along roads, avenues etc. Fl. & Fr.: September-March.

Combination of bark, jaggery, seeds of *Trachyspermum ammi* and *Vernonia cinerea* is given to the animal twice a day upto one month as a tonic to remove overall weakness. Infusion of bark has cooling effect on animal body. Decoction of 2 to 3 years matured thorns is given to the animal for removal of retained placenta after delivery. Pods are given with fodder during pregnancy and after delivery to increase lactation. Decoction of bark is applied over hooves twice a day to treat foot and mouth disease. About 1 Kg. immature pods are given to the animal every morning and evening to increase the lactation. Decoction of stem bark act as antiseptic and applied on wounds.

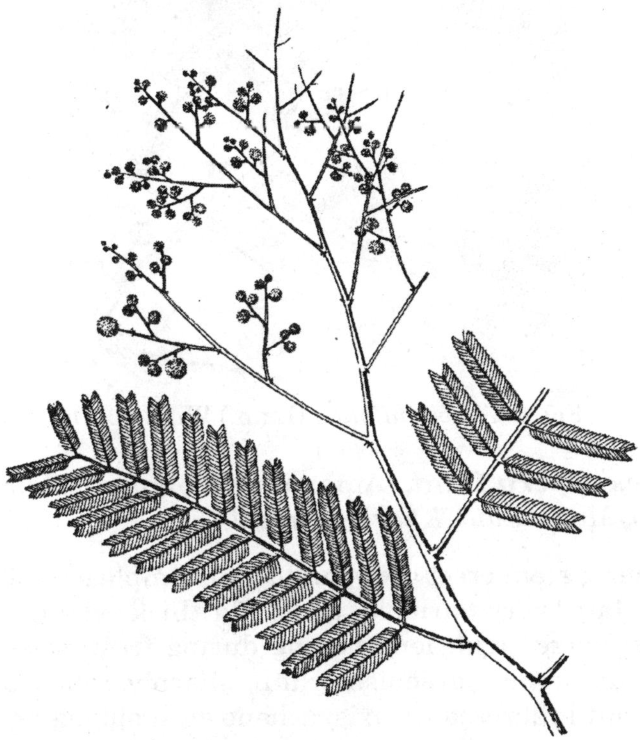

Fig. 4. *Acacia leucophloea* (Roxb.) Willd.

Acacia pennata (Linn.) Willd. (Mimosaceae) *Cheela*

Large, scandent bush or liana with polished bark; prickles slightly recurved; pinnae 8-15 pairs, with glands between the upper ones; leaflets 40-50 pairs; flowers creamy – white or pale – yellow; pods stalked, linear-oblong, glabrous. Rare, in mixed dry deciduous forests. Fl. & Fr.: September-February.

Extract of root bark is given orally once in a day to treat rheumatism.

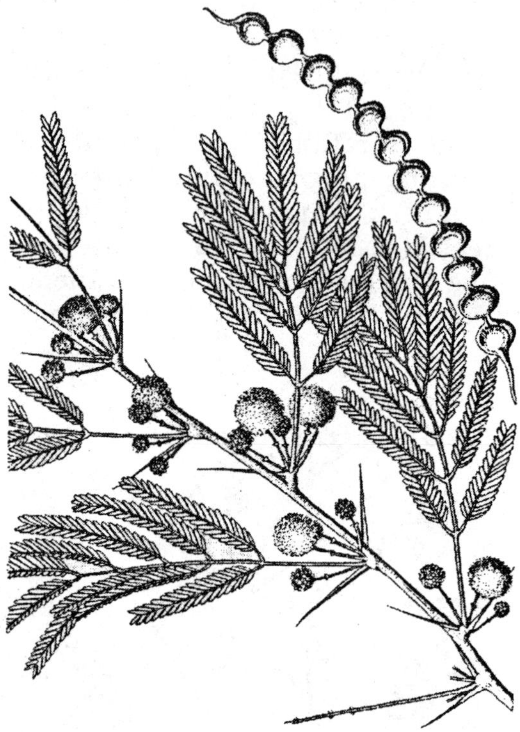

Fig. 5. *Acacia nilotica* (Linn.) Willd. ex Del.

Achyranthes aspera **Linn. (Amaranthaceae)** *Andhijhara, Kanta, Undhokanto, Modokanto, Kharia* (Plate 2)

A stiff herb; stem erect grows upto 1 m, simple or branched; leaves simple, petiolate, very variable, generally thick, young tomentose on both surface; spike rigid, lengthening during fruiting as much as 60 cm; flowers numerous, greenish white, sharply reflexed against the stout pubescent inflorescence axis; achene with oblong or ovate utricle, enclosed in the hardened perianth; seeds oblong brown. Common weed, occur in dry sandy localities. Fl. & Fr.: August- November.

Decoction of about 100 g roots and 50 g rhizomes of *Curcuma longa* prepared in 200 ml urine of child is given to camel to treat stomachache. Half cup of root extract is given to animal to increase lactation. It acts as lactogogue. Root extract is also given to animal as a tonic. Decoction of the whole plant is given for removal of retained placenta after delivery. Leaf extract is used as eye drops for treating opacity of cornea. Seed powder is given to animal to treat dysentery.

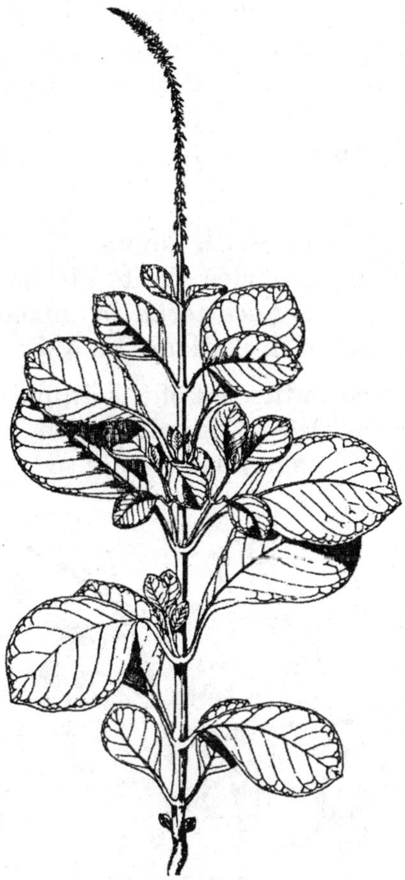

Fig. 6. *Achyranthes aspera* Linn.

Adhatoda zeylanica **Medic. (Acanthaceae)** *Adusa, Aduaa* (Plate 2)

Gregarious shrub, sometimes arborescent, growing upto 7 m. high; leaves simple, petiolate, minutely pubescent; spikes terminal, often several together; flowers bracteate, bracteolate, white, 1.25 cm broad; capsule 1.8 cm long, pubescent, 4 seeded; seeds glabrous. Commonly occurs on foot hills. Fl. & Fr.: October- March.

Extract prepared from the mixture of two to four leaves of this plant, one pod of *Cassia fistula* and five leaves of *Holarrhena antidysenterica,* is given to animal by drenching tube to treat throat infection (*Dhansi*). 100 ml decoction of leaves is given to animal two to three times a day to fever and cough (*Dhansa*) while herbal bath of this is given to animal for removal of ectoparasites and also other skin diseases. Paste prepared from boiled leaves, jaggery and tuber powder of *Curcuma longa* is given orally to treat abscess or septice-mia. Paste prepared from equal amount of bark of *Bombax ceiba* and *Adhadota zeylanica* is given to the animal by drenching tube to treat diarrhoea.

***Aegle marmelos* (Linn.) Corr. (Rutaceae)** *Bel, Bel- patra, Beely* (Plate 2)

Deciduous tree, armed with spines; leaves trifoliate; flowers creamy white in axillary panicles; fruits globose with stony rind and mucilaginous pulp. Sparsely scattered in mixed deciduous forests of the Aravallis; often planted in gardens. Fl. & Fr.: January- July.

The spine is pricked in the tail of the animal for 9 days to treat its degeneration.Poultice of leaves grinded with butter is tied to treat fractured bone. Fruit pulp is applied locally to treat mouth diseases.

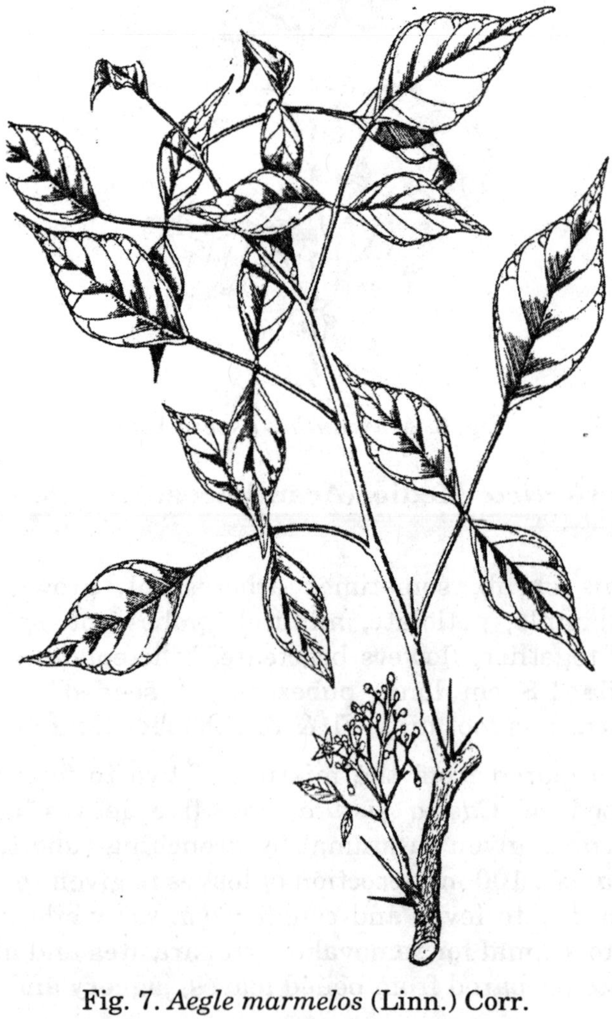

Fig. 7. *Aegle marmelos* (Linn.) Corr.

Aerva lanata **(Linn.) Juss. ex. Schult. (Amaranthaceae)**
Kali Bui, Choti-bui

A small herbaceous plant; leaves suborbicular to lanceolate; flowers bisexual, in axillary spike passing into long leafy inflorescence; fruits rotund, compressed. Mostly in wasteland; locally abundant in arable and fallow fields. Fl. & Fr.: August- March.

Decoction prepared by mixing roots and fruits of *Citrullus colocynthis* is given to the animal to treat constipation. Roots are crushed and given orally as an antidote in snake bite.

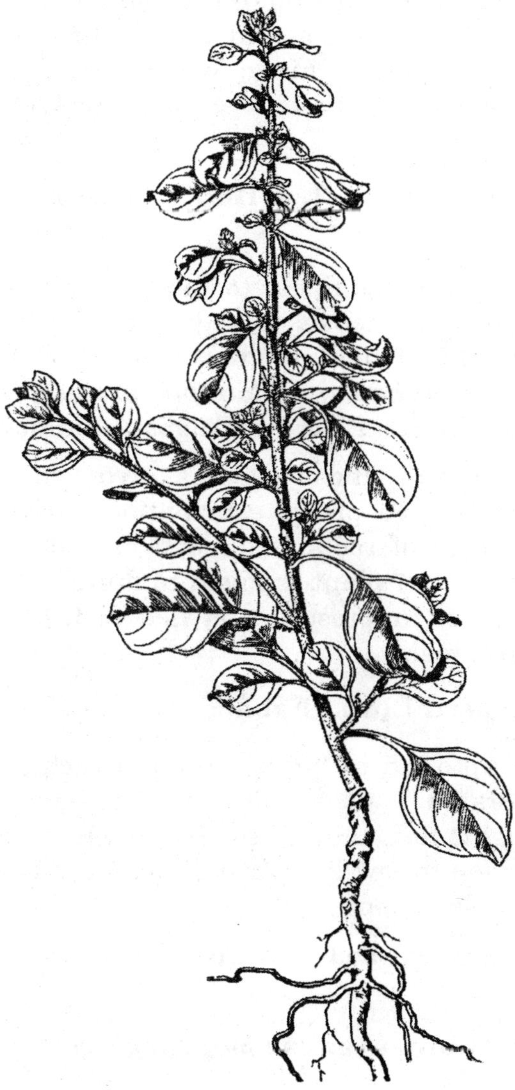

Fig. 8. *Aerva lanata* (Linn.) Juss. ex. Schult.

Aerva javanica **(Burm. f.) Juss. ex Schult (Amaranthaceae)**
Bui, Safed bui

Hairy - tomentose shrub; linear to suborbiular leaves, upto 6 mm broad; flowers woolly, in dense, naked sessile spike; fruits rotund, compressed. Commonly found in gregarious patches in association with *Leptadenia pyrotechnica, Calotropis procera,* and *Saccharum benghalense* on sand dunes.Fl. & Fr.: August –January.

Decoction of flower and leaves is given to the animal to treat digestive disorders and also to promote the discharge of urine in dysuria. Decoction of roots is given orally and paste of roots is applied on foot and mouth to treat foot and mouth disease. Extract of the whole plant is given to the animal when he/she start eating soil. Decoction of inflorescence is used to wash hooves of animal to treat foot and mouth disease.

Aerva pseudotomentosa **Blatt. & Hall. (Amaranthaceae)**
Bui, Safed bui

Hairy - tomentose shrub; linear to suborbicular leaves, upto 6 mm broad; flowers woolly, in dense, naked sessile spike; fruits rotund, compressed. Commonly found in gregarious patches in association with *Leptadenia pyrotechnica, Calotropis procera,* and *Saccharum benghalense* on sand dunes. Fl. & Fr.: August – January.

Decoction of flowers and leaves is given to animal to treat digestive disorders and to promote urination. Decoction of roots is given orally and paste of roots is applied on foot to treat foot and mouth disease. Extract of plant is given to animal when he/she start eating soil. Poultice of inflorescence is tied to treat swelling due to muscular injury in camel.

Aeschynomene aspera **Linn. (Fabaceae)** *Dhadoom*

Annual herb, upto 1.5 m high; stem and rachis of leaves warty; leaves long, flowers in 1 to 4 - flowered, axillary, viscid racemes, yellow; pods straight, flat, muricated, indented on the lower suture; seeds black.. Common in low-lying areas, near ponds and in rice field. Fl. & Fr.: August – November.

Mature pods are crushed and given to cows and buffaloes for oestrus induction.

Agave americana **Linn. (Agavaceae)** *Jangli-gawar-patha* (Plate 2)

Perennial herb with rhizome; leaves simple, alternate, large densely crowded in massive rosettes, thick, fleshy, coated with wax, apex spiny; flowers come after many (5 to 68 sometime 100) years of existence; gigantic racemose or paniculate inflorescence with ultimate branches of few- flowered cymes; flowers large, showy, bisexual; capsule oblong- clavate, beaked. Wild; xerophyte. Fl. & Fr.: Almost throughout the year.

Paste of the leaves is applied over broken horns for early healing.

***Ageratum conyzoides* Linn. (Asteraceae)** *Tokariyo*

Erect hairy, annual herb; leaves ovate or rhomboid-ovate, triangular; head in terminal corymbs; achenes 1.5-1.8 mm long, angled, black; pappus - scales serrate, awn - tipped. Common in wet and shady habitats from plains to hills, often gregarious in orchards. Fl. & Fr.: Throughout the year.

The poultice of whole plant is tied over boil and wound as an antiseptic.

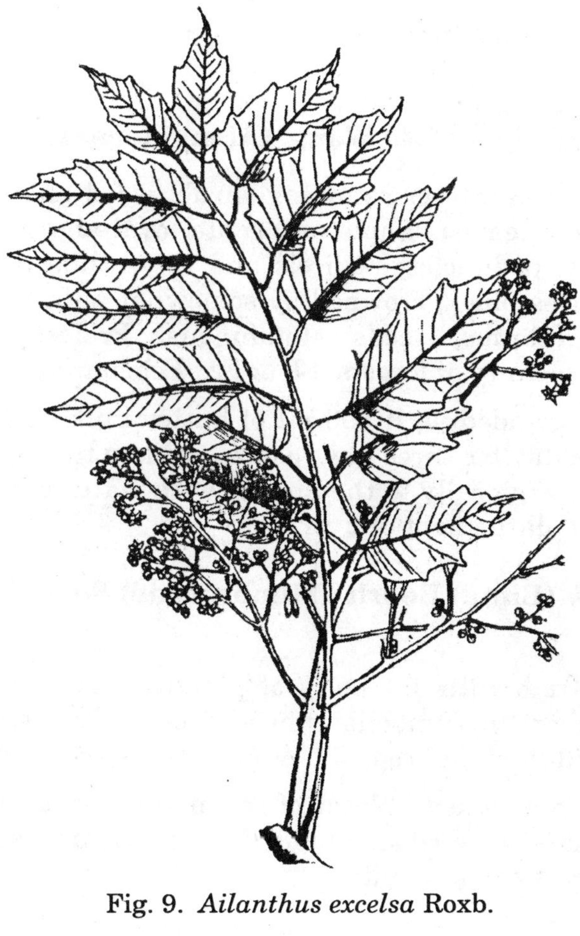

Fig. 9. *Ailanthus excelsa* Roxb.

***Ailanthus excelsa* Roxb. (Simroubaceae)** *Arru, Ardu*

Large trees; with pinnate leaves crowded at the end of branches; flowers yellow, in terminal and axillary panicles; fruit samara, spindle shaped, 1-seeded. Planted mostly along road sides and on field boundaries. Fl. & Fr.: February- May.

Bark extract is given to animals by drenching tube to treat flatulence. Extract of bark is also given to animals orally twice a day for three days to treat asthma, bronchitis and pneumonia. Leaf decoction (250 ml) is given orally to treat fever.

***Alternanthera pungens* Kunth (Amaranthaceae)** *Kuttiya*

Prostrate perennial herb; leaves rhomboid - ovate to broadly ovate; flowers axillary; seeds rounded, faintly reticulate. Widespread as a weed, along road sides, railway tracks. Fl. & Fr.: Almost throughout the year.

Decoction of whole plant is rubbed over the animal body to remove lice and ticks.

***Alangium salvifolium* (L.f.) Wang. (Alangiaceae)** *Aankol, Ankola*

Small deciduous tree or rambling shrub; wood olive brown, hard and close grained; leaves simple, alternate, ovate-lanceolate; flowers in close fascicles, peduncles, pedicels and calyx tube usually woolly, silky white, berries black, crowned by somewhat enlarged calyx-limb, pubescent or glabrous; seeds albuminous. Prefers dry climate; profusely in the vicinity of forests. Fl. & Fr.: February-June.

50 g root is grinded with 500 ml of butter milk and given to the animal once in a day for three days as an antidote to dog bite. Paste of 100 g leaves is given orally to the animal with water to treat malarial fever as well as enlargement of liver.

***Albizia lebbeck* (Linn.) Benth. (Mimosaceae)** *Siris, Saras, Siras* (Plate 2)

Deciduous tree; with 1-4 pairs of pinnae, 4-10 pairs of leaflets; flowers pale green, in umbellate heads; pods flat, straw-coloured. Frequently found in plain areas. Fl. & Fr.: August-December.

Milk of sheep is mixed in latex of this plant and used as eye drops to treat conjunctivitis. Tribals claim that it can be used by human beings also to treat conjunctivitis.

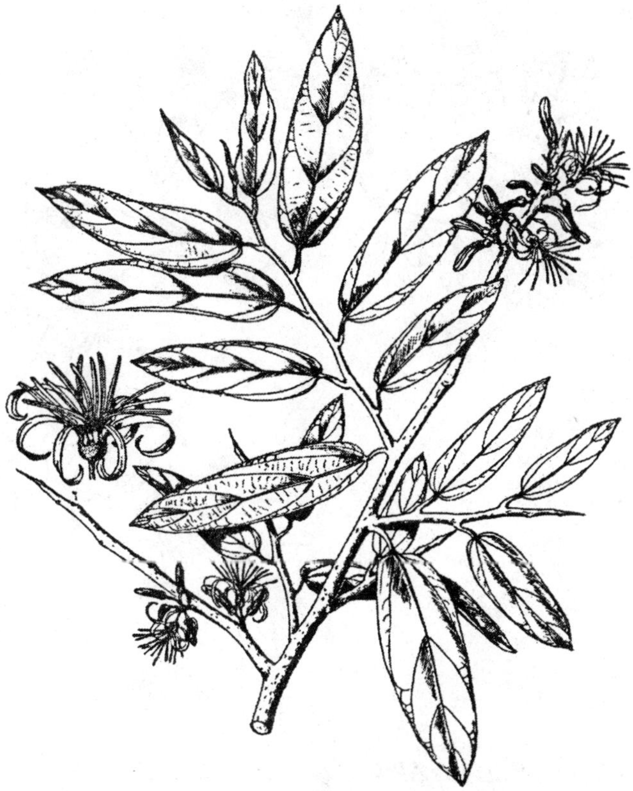

Fig. 10. *Alangium salvifolium* (L.f.) Wang.

***Allium cepa* Linn. (Liliaceae)** *Kanda, Pyaj*

Scapigerous annual herbs; leaves fistular; flowers white in umbels. Commonly cultivated for its underground stem (bulb) used as vegetable. Fl. & Fr.: October – January.

To overcome the calcium deficiency and overall weakness after delivery, bulbs of *Allium cepa* are fed to the cattle.

***Allium sativum* Linn. (Liliaceae)** *Lahsan*

Bulbose herbs; bulb short, bulblets or cloves fleshy, creamy yellow, ovoid, acuminate; leaves 15 – 30 cm long; flowers white, in umbels. Commonly cultivated as winter crop. Fl. & Fr.: August – October.

Paste of 250 g single tillered bulbs is mixed with two eggs of hen and 1 litre of milk and given to the animal to treat impaction and lumbago. Bulbs of *Allium sativum* are boiled in seed oil of *Brassica campestris,* cooled it and given orally to the animal to treat weakness, foot and mouth disease and impaction.

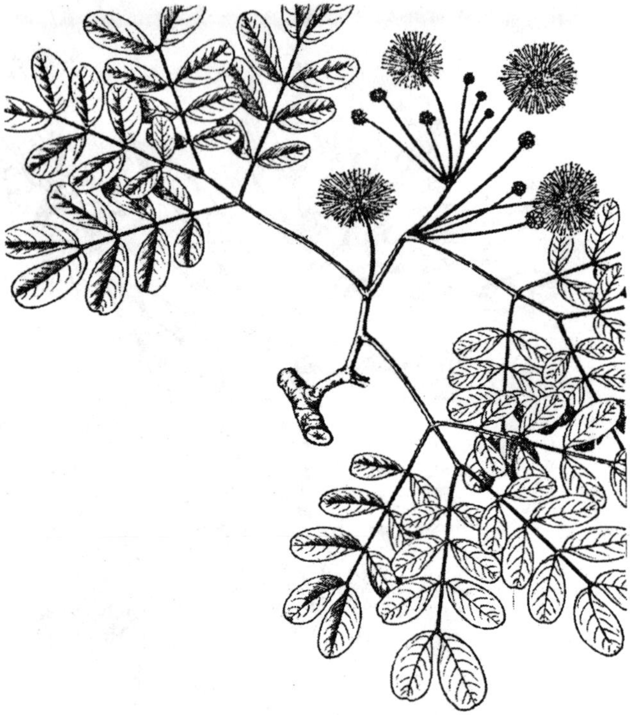

Fig. 11. *Albizia lebbeck* (Linn.) Benth.

***Aloe vera* Linn. (Liliaceae)** *Gawarpatha*

A coarse looking plant with a short (30 - 60 cm high) stem; leaves succulent, green, large, densely crowded; flowers in racemes, bright yellow, tubular, stamens frequently projected beyond the perianth tube. Common in burial places, where it is invariably grown on the graves by muslims. Fl. & Fr.: October – March.

Pulp of leaves is applied to treat skin irritation, burns and inflammation.

***Amaranthus spinosus* Linn. (Amaranthaceae)** *Chouli, Chawli, Adak dhatura*

Erect, annual herb, upto 60 cm in height; stem green, woody, glabrous, branched, armed with prickles; leaves simple, axils with 5 spines; spike axillary, usually densely flowered; unisexual; seeds very small, black, shining. Grows wild or semi wild, preferably in waste-lands. Fl. & Fr.: Throughout the year.

The whole plant is fed to the animals as galactagogue.

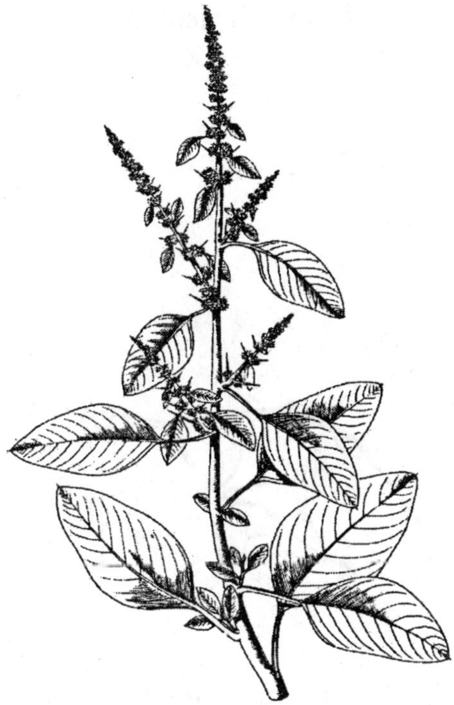

Fig. 12. *Amaranthus spinosus* Linn.

***Ampelocissus latifolia* (Roxb.) Planch.(Vitaceae)** *Khata nimbu* (Plate 3)

Climber, tendrils leaf opposed, stem weak hollow, glabrous; leaves alternate, petiolate, simple; cymes compact, densely woolly, peduncle long, stout, woody, peduncle bears a long wiry forked tendril below the cyme; fruits black, 2- seeded. Grows in hilly terrain; wild. Fl. & Fr.: July- October.

About 50 g tubers are crushed and given to the animal with water, twice a day for three days to treat the fractured bone. This extract is also given to animals by drenching tube to treat flatulence. Extract of aerial part is given orally to animals by drenching tube to treat bronchitis.

***Anacardium occidentale* Linn. (Anacardiaceae)** *Kaju*

Spreading evergreen perennial tree to 12 m tall; leaves simple, alternate, obovate, glabrous; flowers numerous in terminal panicles, 10–20 cm long, male or female, green and reddish, radially symmetrical nearly; fruit a reniform achene, about 3 cm long, 2.5 cm wide, called the cashew-apple. Fl. & Fr.: January – May.

Latex is applied to treat the foot disease and as antiseptic on wound.

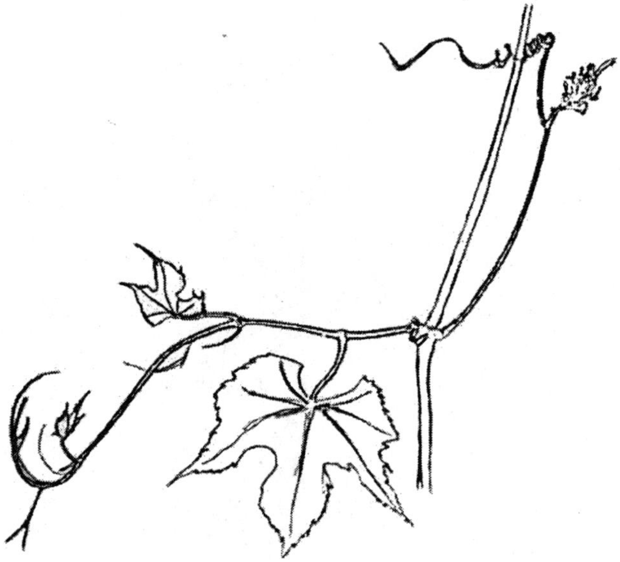

Fig. 13. *Ampelocissus latifolia* (Roxb.) Planch

Anethum graveolens **Linn. (Apiaceae)** *Suwa*

Annual or biennial herb; stem erect, slightly grooved; leaves alternate, light green, decompounded, contain oil; flowers in compound umbel; fruits brown, oval, dry, grooved, consist of 2 compressed, indehiscent parts, winged, odour and taste characteristically aromatic. Plant of cold climate, grows well in good garden soil. Fl. & Fr.: August – January.

Milch- cattle are fed with porridge prepared from seeds of this plant seeds of *Trigonella foenum-graecum* and *Triticum aestivum* as a galactagogue. Powder of seeds is given orally to the animals in vulvo-vaginal- uterine- prolapse.

Anisomeles indica **(Linn.) O. Kuntz (Lamiaceae)** *Phulmajri, Gobariya*

A small, smelling, softly pubescent herb, 90-180 cm high, sparingly hairy or densely pubescent; leaves ovate, acute or obtuse to sub-acuminate, crenate-serrate, rounded-cordate to cuneate at base; flowers sessile, in dense axillary whorls, combined into terminal dense spikes, bluish- purple. Occurs in wastelands and scrub- jungles. Fl. & Fr.: August-December.

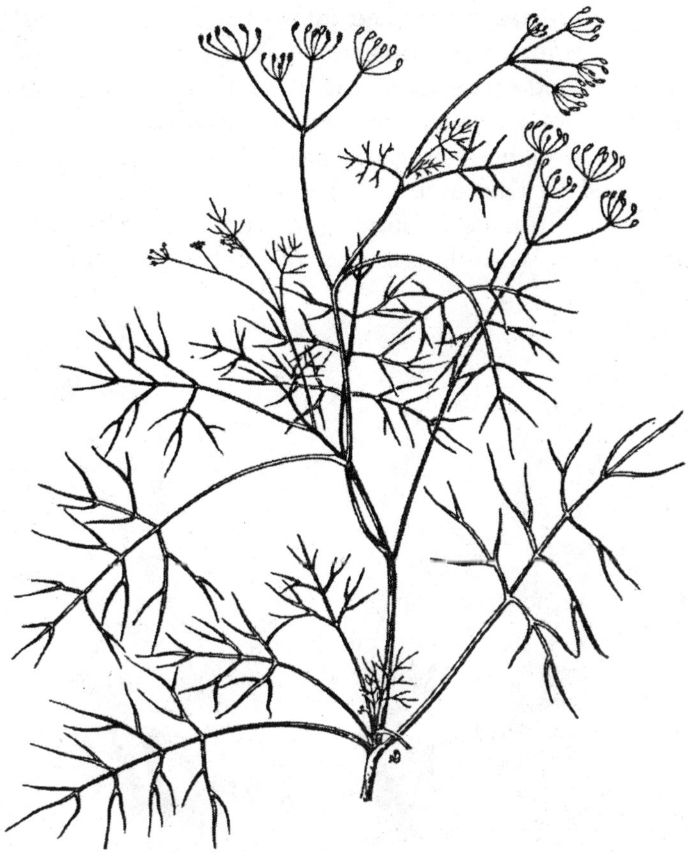

Fig. 14. *Anethum graveolens* Linn.

Extract of whole plant is given to animals to treat indigestion. Decoction of the plant is given to buffaloes to treat flatulence and leucorrhoea. There is a belief that if animals suffering from foot and mouth disease pass across this plant, they become well. Extract of stem is given to animals to treat indigestion.

***Annona squamosa* Linn. (Annonaceae)** *Sitaphal, Anduri* (Plate 3)

Evergreen shrub or small tree; with oblong- lanceolate leaves, nearly glabrous and slightly scented; flowers drooping, yellowish green; fruits globose or ovoid with projecting areoles. Naturalized in the valleys and along streams throughout the Aravalli range. Fl. & Fr.: April- August.

Paste of 100 g leaves is given to the animal with fodder to treat constipation. Five to seven leaves are grinded with a pinch of Sodium carbonate, a pinch of resin of *Ferula asafoetida* and mixed with 200 to 400g oil of *Sesamum indicum* or *Arachis hypogaea* or *Ricinus comm-*

unis or *Linum usitatissimum* and given to the animal with drenching tube or bottle to remove the internal parasites. Dosage of this preparation depends on body weight of the animal. Leaf paste is applied over the infected part of the body to remove external parasites. Paste of leaves is applied over hooves of animal to treat foot and mouth disease. It is also sprayed in the shed of animal as a disinfectant. The injured part of cows and buffaloes is bandaged with the leaves of this plant for early healing of the wounds. Extract of bark is given to animals orally to treat bronchitis.

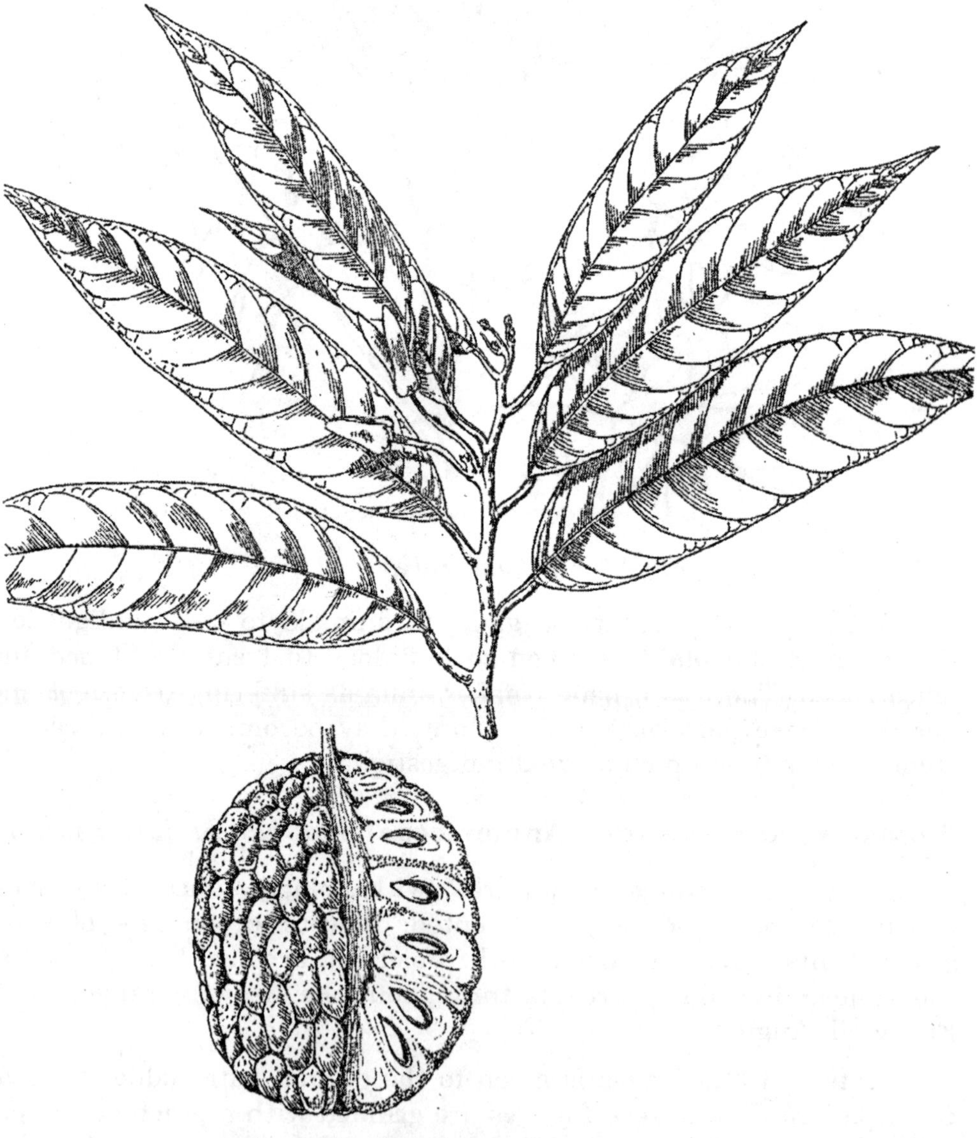

Fig. 15. *Annona squamosa* Linn.

Anogeissus latifolia **(Roxb. ex DC.) Wall. ex Guill. & Perr. (Combretaceae)** *Dhokada, Dhavada*

Usually small tree, leafless during most of the hot season; trunk erect, branchlets drooping, bark whitish grey, smooth, having shallow, irregular depression; leaves alternate or apparently opposite; flowers in dense, globose heads on axillary peduncles. Common in mixed dry deciduous forests associated with *Anogeissus pendula.* Fl. & Fr.: September- March.

Extract prepared from 100 g powdered bark is given to animal twice a day for two days to get relief from fever.

Apluda mutica **Linn. (Poaceae)** *Bhangto, Tamta bheda*

Annuals; leaves linear-lanceolate, long acuminate, base narrowed; ligule membranous, rounded; panicles of 2 to many, simple racemes terminating the culms, enclosed in a peduncled spathe; spikelets in three, one sessile and two pedicelled; seeds caryopsis. Common on the hills, among hedges of cultivated field and bushes in wastelands preferring moist places. Fl. & Fr.: August- February.

Whole plant is fed to the animal as antidote against insect-bite. Paste of whole plant is used to treat mouth sores of cattle.

Argemone mexicana **Linn. (Papaveraceae)** *Satyanashi, Dholari*

A prickly herb; 60 - 90 cm with yellow latex; leaves sinuate, pinnatifid, green and white, half amplexicaul; flowers 50 mm in diameter, yellow, sepals cuspidate; capsules 20 - 38 mm long. Growing gregariously in open - waste places. A troublesome weed for both Kharif and Rabi crops. Fl. & Fr.: February – June.

Leaf extract is applied locally on wounds and boils as antiseptic. Latex is applied externally to treat various skin diseases.

Argyreia nervosa **(Burm. f.) Bojer (Convolvulaceae)** *Samandar-bel*

White tomentose, large twiner; with ovate-cordate leaves which are glabrous above and tomentose beneath; flowers rose - purple and white, in subcapitate cymes. Cultivated in the gardens for large handsome foliage and beautiful flowers. Fl. & Fr.: September-January.

Poultice of leaves is tied over neck to treat tonsillitis in animals. Leaf extract is applied locally on wound.

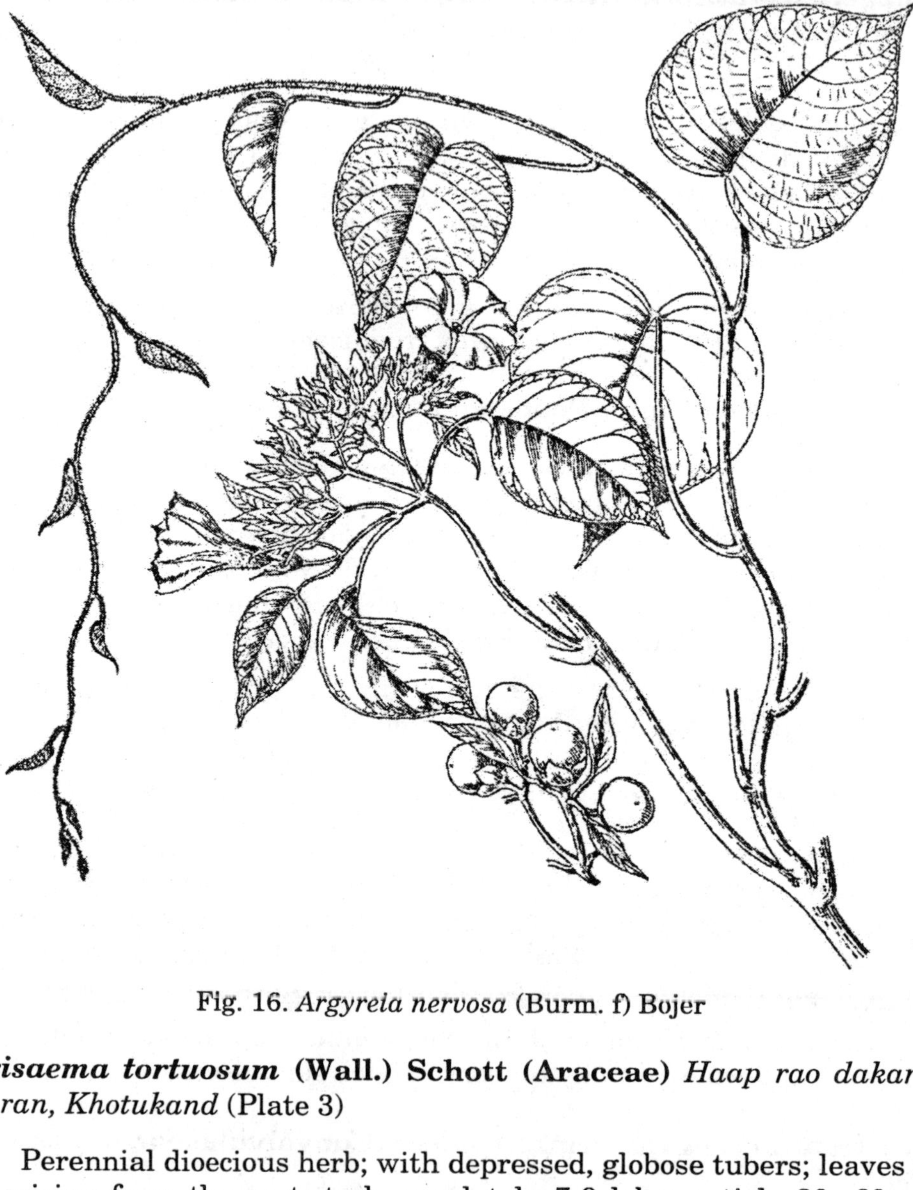

Fig. 16. *Argyreia nervosa* (Burm. f) Bojer

***Arisaema tortuosum* (Wall.) Schott (Araceae)** *Haap rao dakaro, Suran, Khotukand* (Plate 3)

Perennial dioecious herb; with depressed, globose tubers; leaves 2-3, arising from the root-stock, pendately 7-9 lobe; petiole 20- 60 cm long, spadix curved or sigmoid; spathes greenish; fruits ovoid, red. Rare, in shady localities in the gardens, ravine slopes and forest edges. Fl. & Fr.: July-August.

Decoction of tuber is given to animals through drenching tube to treat. flatulence, and other gastric disorders. Fresh tuber is crushed and given to domestic animals along with green fodder to treat fractured bone.

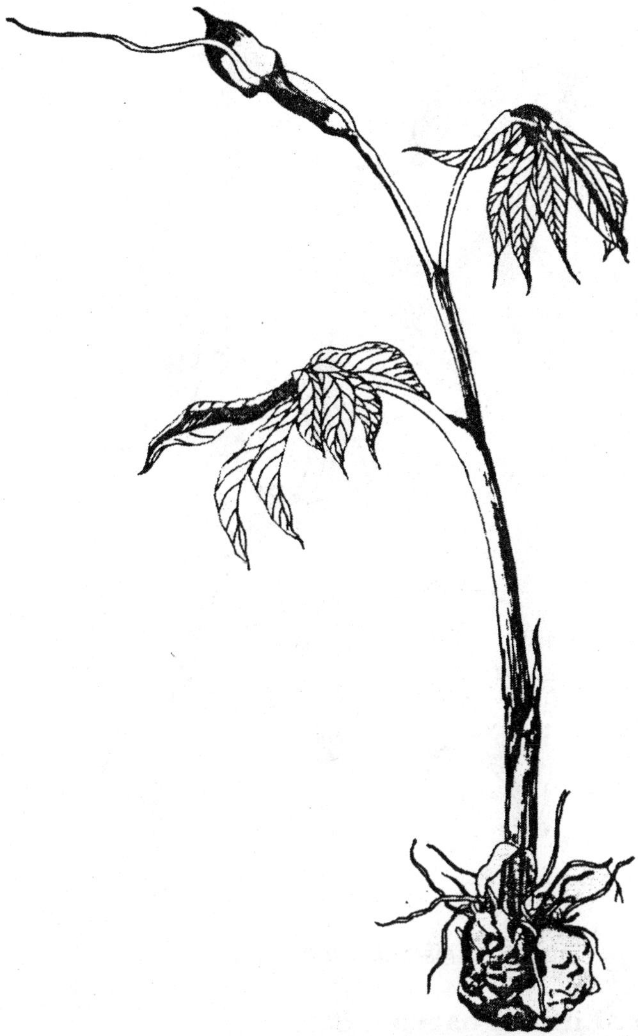

Fig. 17. *Arisaema tortuosum* (Wall.) Schott

***Aristolochia bracteolata* Lam. (Aristolochiaceae)** *Kadhu, Kalipad* (Plate 3)

Prostrate bitter herb; root perennial; stem slender, decumbent, angled, striate; leaves petiolate, reniform or broadly cordate, glaucous beneath; peduncle bracteate; flower solitary, tubular with globose base, villous nearly 2.5 cm long; fruit pyriform, many seeded; seeds triangular. Common in wastelands, along with river banks and paddy fields. Fl. & Fr.: August- September.

About 10 g root is given with bread of wheat, thrice in a day upto 4 days to treat fever. Leaf decoction is given orally to treat arthritis.

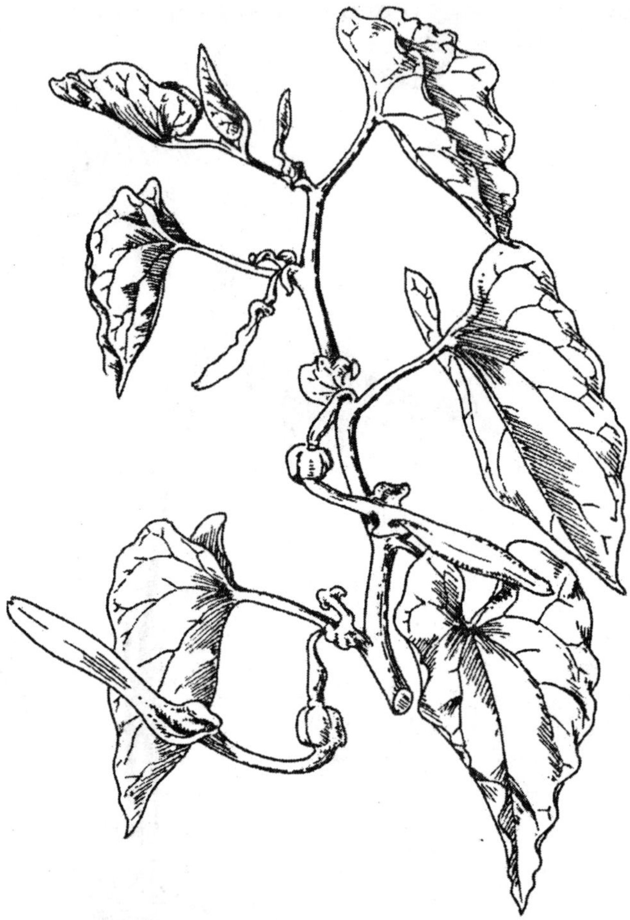

Fig. 18. *Aristolochia bracteolata* Lam.

Arundo donax* Linn. (Poaccac) *Baru

Erect, stout, tall, perennial grass, upto 2.5 m high, with creeping woody rhizome; culms fistular; leaves 15 - 50 by 2 - 5 cm, distichous, linear - lanceolate; spikelets 1- 1.5 cm long, light brown, 2 – flowered; fruits caryopsis with linear hilum. Commonly found in marshy habitats along the rivers and streams, particularly in dried up beds. Fl. & Fr.: August – October.

Decoction of rhizome is given orally to treat dysentery.

***Asparagus racemosus* Willd. (Liliaceae)** *Satawari* (Plate 3)

A slender, scrambling/ scandent suffruticose perennial, woody, prickly shoots with reflexed spines; cladode more or less acicular and triquetrous falcate, 13 - 26 mm long; divaricate, finely acuminate;

flowers white, sweet-scented, 6 mm on filiform articulate pedicels, 6 - 12 mm long in very short racemes; berries 2.5 - 6 mm in diameter, scarlet red on ripening. Frequently found along with hedge in plains and hilly areas. Fl. & Fr.: November- January.

Milch – animal is fed with whole plant of *Asparagus racemosus* early in the morning with empty stomach to increase the secretion of milk. Paste of stem is applied on broken horn for early healing.

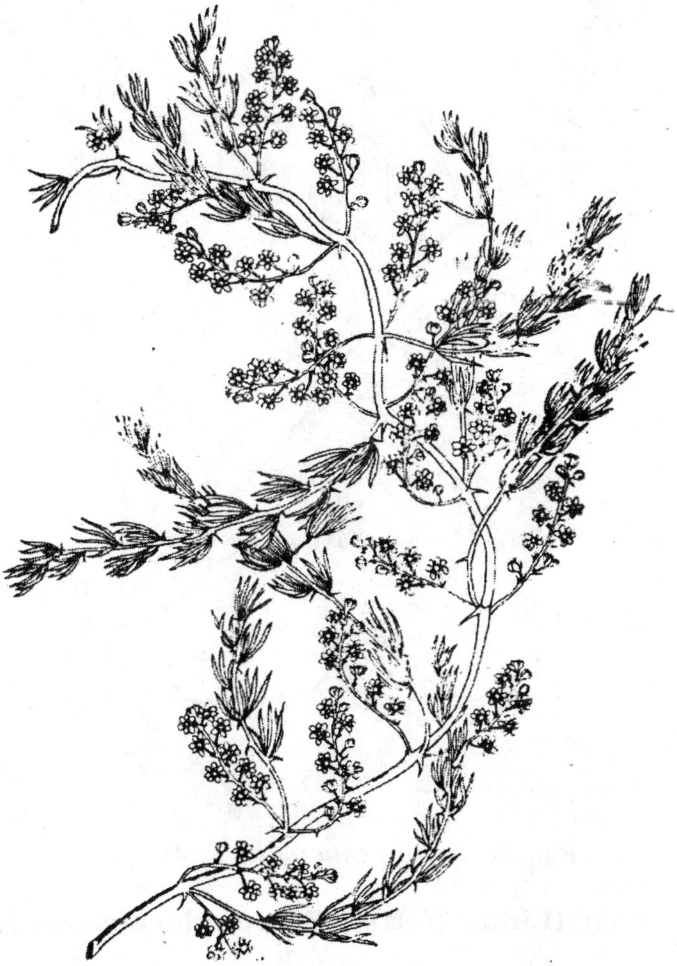

Fig. 19. *Asparagus racemosus* Willd.

***Azadirachta indica* A. Juss. (Meliaceae)** *Neemda, Neemoda, Limbada, Neemdi*

Evergreen tree, 12-17 m high, trunk straight, bark brownish black, longitudinally fissured; leaves crowded at the ends of branches;

petiole 6 cm long; leaflets subopposite; bracts caducous, ovate-lanceolate; panicles axillary. Thrives best in drier climate with normal temperature not exceeding 40°C and rainfall varying from 45 to 112 cm/year, prefers black- cotton soil though grows on all kind of soils. Fl. & Fr.: March- July.

Leaves of *Azadirachta indica* are given as fodder to the animals to treat leucorrhoea.

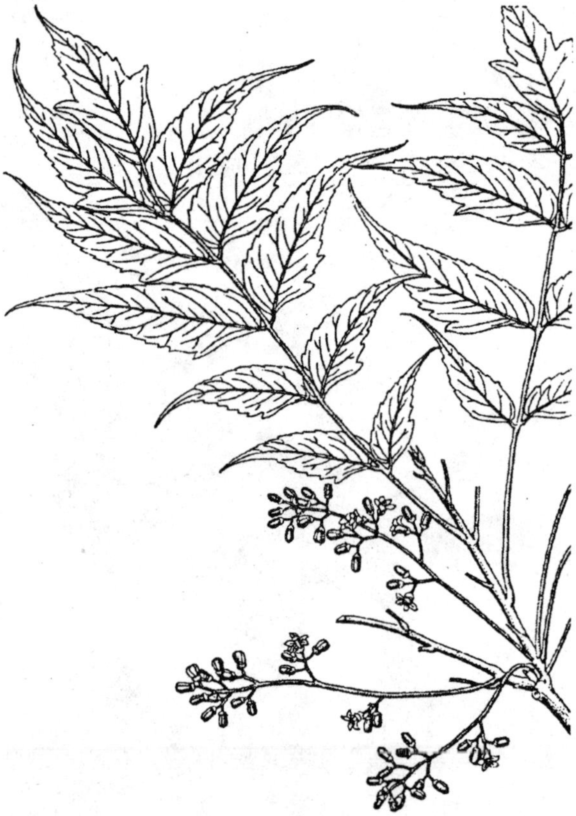

Fig. 20. *Azadirachta indica* A. Juss.

Bacopa monnieri (Linn.) Wettst. (Scrophulariaceae) *Brahmi, Baam*

Annual creeper, rooting at each node; stem soft, succulent, soft hairs present; leaves alternate, simple, sessile or subsessile, oval shaped; flowers 0.8-1.5 cm long; capsule 2-grooved, valves separating from entire column, many seeded. Grows in damp or marshy areas, on the banks of ponds, canals and crop fields. Fl. & Fr.: Throughout the year.

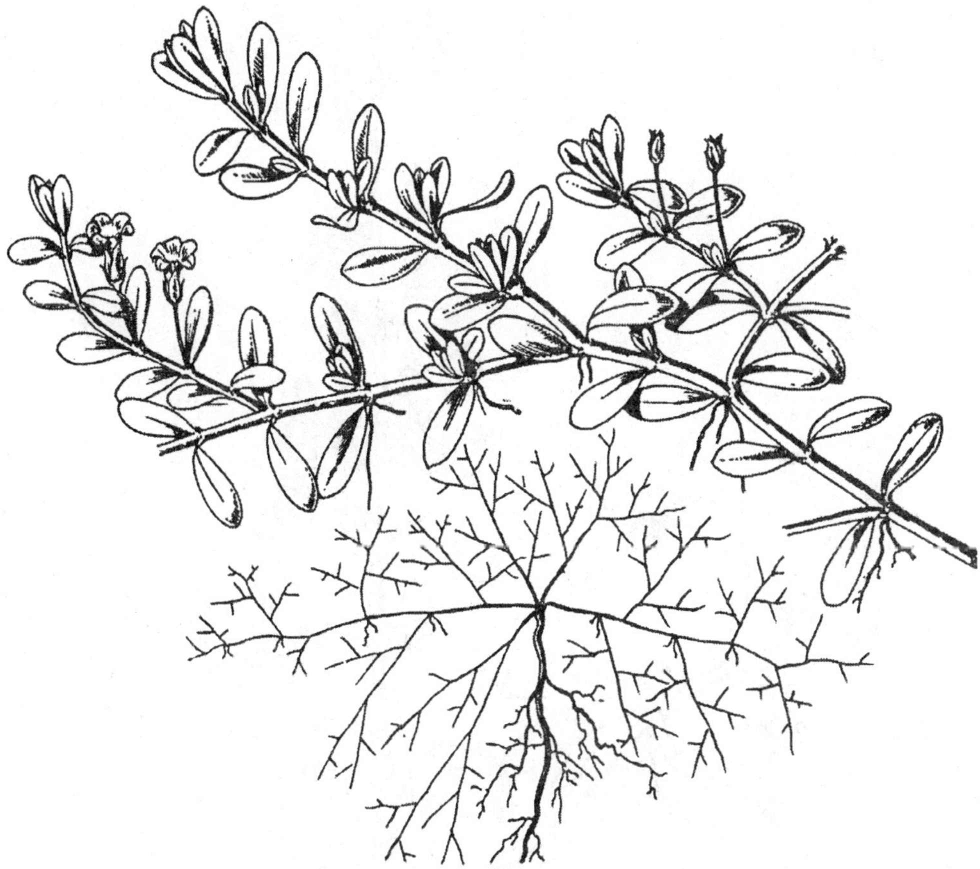

Fig. 21. *Bacopa monnieri* (Linn.) Wettst.

Paste of whole plant of *Bacopa monnieri* is given to the animal to treat paralytic attack. A single dose is sufficient.

***Balanites aegyptiaca* (Linn.) Delile (Balanitaceae)** *Hingor, Hingul, Hingota, Hingora, Hingot*

Spiny tree, about 6 m high; branches glabrous or puberulous and ending in very strong ascending spines; leaves alternate, trifoliate, ashy green, leaflets coriaceous; cymes axillary, 4 to 10 flowered, flowers green, velvety pubescent; fruit ovoid, about 5 cm in length, fleshy drupes, 1 seeded; seed oily but exalbuminous. Xerophyte, found chiefly on black cotton soil; does not thrive in rocky areas. Fl. & Fr.: February – May.

Stem bark is powdered and given to the cattle to increase the secretion of milk. It is also given to treat intestinal worms. Paste of bark is given orally to animals in snake-bite as antidote.

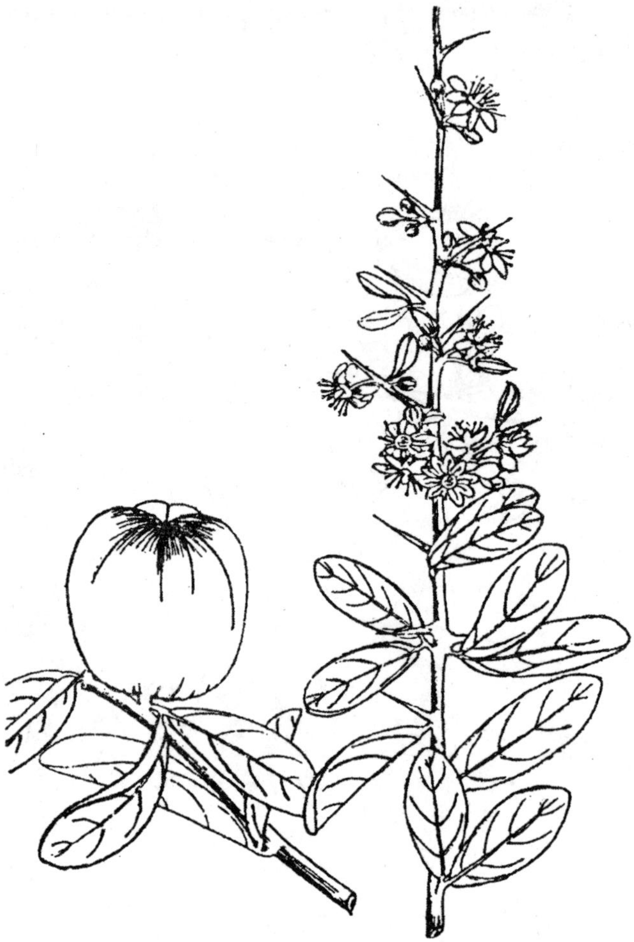

Fig. 22. *Balanites aegyptiaca* (Linn.) Delile

***Barleria prionitis* Linn. (Acanthaceae)** *Bajradanti, Kanta sulio* (Plate 3)

Unarmed undershrub; leaves elliptic-oblong; yellow flowers in dense spikes, calyx-lobes glandular; capsules 4- seeded. Common grows on hilly tracts. Fl. & Fr.: August- November.

Paste of leaves is applied locally on skin to treat eczema and itching.

***Bauhinia purpurea* Linn. (Caesalpiniaceae)** *Khata hatra*

Shrub or small tree; leaves suborbicular; flowers in terminal racemes; pods linear, flat, apiculate, reddish brown. Commonly planted in the gardens and along the roads. Fl. & Fr.: May – November.

Decoction of stem bark is given to treat swelling of neck. Decoction is also given to treat fractured bone.

***Bauhinia racemosa* Lam. (Caesalpiniaceae)** *Jhinjha*

Small tree, with drooping branches; leaves simple, deeply 2-lobed; flowers white, in terminal or leaf-opposed racemes; pods slightly falcate. Grows in the hilly tracts and plains. Fl. & Fr.: April - July.

Extract of leaves is given orally to treat diarrhoea. Paste of stem bark is applied locally to treat wound.

***Bauhinia variegata* Linn. (Caesalpiniaceae)** *Kachnar*

Small to medium-sized deciduous tree: leaves minute stipules 1-2 mm, early caducous; flower racemes unbranched at ends of twigs; pods dehiscent, strap-shaped, obliquely striate, 20-30 by 2-2.5 cm; seeds brown, flat, nearly circular with coriaceous testa. Planted as an ornamental tree on account of its beautiful flower. Fl. & Fr.: February – April.

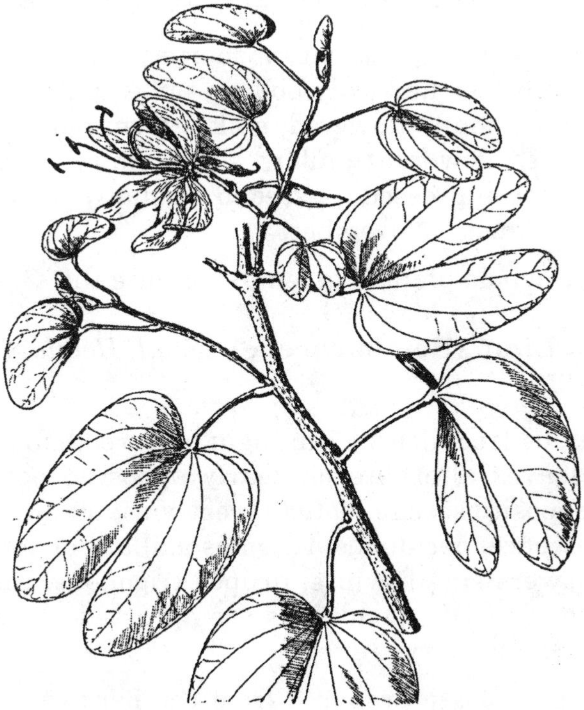

Fig. 23. *Bauhinia variegata* Linn.

Luke warm decoction of bark is used to wash wound of foot and mouth disease.

Bidens biternata **(Lour.) Merr. & Sherff ex Sherff (Asteraceae)**
Samara Kodaki

Erect annual herb; leaves 1- pinnate; heads 10 -30 flowered, solitary, pedunculate, yellow; ray florets ligulate, neuter or female; disk florets tubular, bisexual; achenes 0.5 - 2.0 cm long, linear, glabrous, black; pappus 2-4, rigid, retrorsely hispid, awned. Natura-lized in the forests from plains to the hills. Fl. & Fr.: August – January.

Decoction of whole plant is given orally to increases the secretion of milk and applied locally on cut and wounds as antiseptic.

Biophytum sensitivum **(Linn.) DC. (Oxalidaceae)** *Lajwanti*

Erect annual herb; stem clothed with appressed or erecto-patent hairs; leaves with 3-12 pairs of leaflets; flowers yellow; capsule subglobose, apiculate, stellately 5 - valved. Rare, in the forests and gardens in shady habitats. Fl. & Fr.: September – October.

Extract of leaves is applied locally for healing of cut and wounds.

Blepharis linariaefolia **Pers. (Acanthaceae)** *Unt-kantilo*

Rigid herb; stem 7.5 - 15 cm or shorter; leaves opposite or in a whorl, simple, linear or narrowly oblong, pubescent, toothed or spinescent; heads few or many flowered; spikes terminal or on suppressed axillary branches; flowers tubular, softly hairy; capsules shining brown, ellipsoid, compressed, 2-seeded. Usually found on gravelly soils. Fl. & Fr.: August – November.

Decoction of whole plant is given to increase the secretion of milk.

Bombax ceiba **Linn. (Bombacaceae)** *Semal, Hemlo, Heembal, Sanwal* (Plate 3)

Balsamiferous tree, nearly 7 m high; bark reddish or grey, peeling off in flakes; leaves alternate or nearly opposite, petiolate, imparipinnate with opposite sessile leaflets, very variable in size, shape and degree of pubescence, deciduous, racemes axillary or terminal, shorter than leaves; flowers small, white; drupes trigonous, containing three 1-seeded pyrenes; seeds pendulous, compressed. Very common in forests. Fl. & Fr.: February- June.

The poultice of paste prepared from the bark of *Bombax ceiba* is tied around fractured bone and then *Bambusa arundinacea* strips are tied with the help of fallen human hairs dipped in mustard (*Brassica campestris*) oil. Flowers of *Bombax ceiba* are mixed with fodder and given to animal for disposal of placenta after delivery. Flowers of *Bombax ceiba* are mixed with the powdered stem bark of *Alangium salvifolium* and given to the animals for the disposal of placenta after delivery. The flowers are kept in an earthen pot filled with water for whole night and sugar is mixed in this infusion and candy is prepared and given orally to animals to treat urinary disorders.

***Boswellia serrata* Roxb. ex Colebr. (Burseraceae)** *Salar, Halar*

Balsamiferous tree, nearly 7 m high; bark dark reddish or grey, peeling off in flakes; leaves alternate or nearly opposite, petiolate, imparipinnate with opposite sessile leaflets, vary variable in size, shape and degree of pubescence, deciduous; raceme axillary or terminal, shorter than leaves; flowers small, white; drupes trigonous, containing three 1-seeded pyrenes; seeds pendulous, compressed. Very common in forests, abundant on Aravalli hills in mixed dry deciduous forests. Fl. & Fr.: April - December.

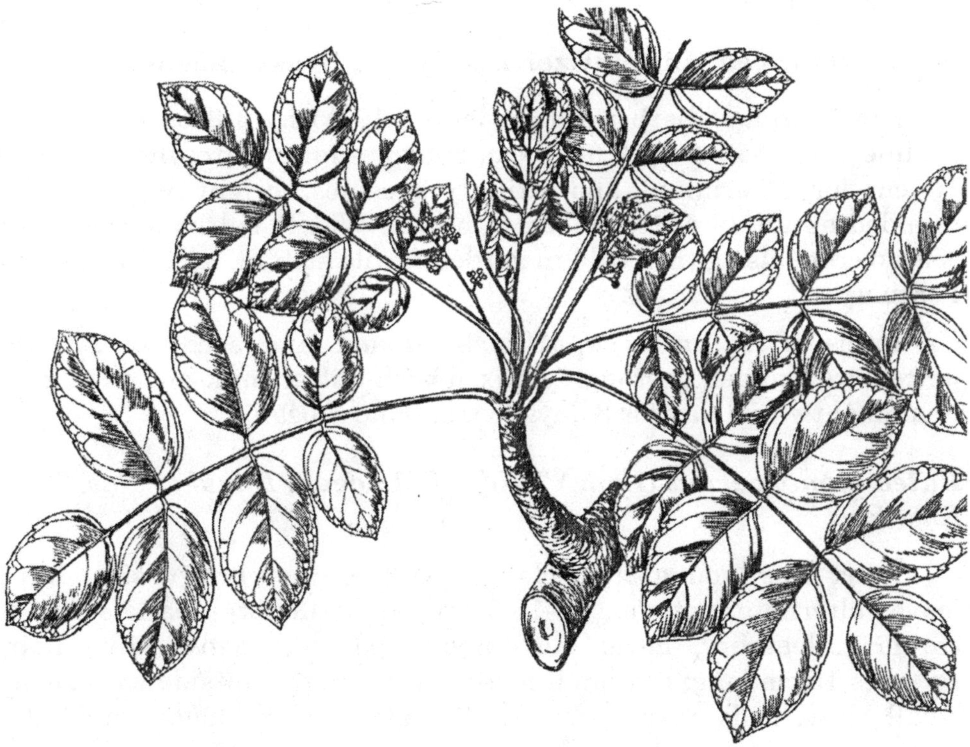

Fig. 24. *Boswellia serrata* Roxb. ex Cocls.

Decoction of stem bark is given to animals to treat arthritis and digestive disorders (indigestion, windiness and flatulence). Infusion of 2 kg powdered bark is divided in three equal doses and each dose is given orally to animal early in the morning to dissolve iron piece engulfed by the animal accidentally.

***Brassica campestris* Linn. (Brassicaceae)** *Sarson*

Annual erect herb; radical leaves 20-30 by 3-5 cm; cauline ones 3-6 by 1-2 cm; flower in terminal raceme, yellow; seeds minute, glabrous, yellowish-brown. Extensively cultivated as a winter season crop for the edible oil obtained from the seeds. Fl. & Fr.: January – April.

A pinch of *Ferula asafoetida* (hing) mixed with 500 ml oil of *Brassica campestris* is given to the animal with the help of drenching tube to treat indigestion and flatulence. 'Sindoor' (vermilion, red lead) is mixed with few drops of oil of *Brassica campestris* and applied on broken horn for early healing. Sulphur is mixed with oil of *Brassica campestris* and applied on the body of animal to all kinds of skin diseases.

***Brassica juncea* (Linn.) Czern. & Coss. (Brassicaceae)** *Rai*

Erect, annual herbs; radical leaves 10-25 by 4-8 cm, pinnatifid, cauline ones 3.5-8.0 by 2.0-3.5 cm, oblong – lanceolate; flowers in 10-15 cm long, terminal and axillary recemes, bright yellow; seeds rounded minutely pitted, blackish brown. Widely cultivated as a cold season crop; also grows wild in garden fertile soil. Fl. & Fr.: December-February.

Bulbs of *Allium cepa, Allium sativum* and seeds of *Brassica juncea* are grinded thoroughly mixed with butter milk and then given to animal twice a day for 3 days to treat diarrhoea.

***Butea monosperma* (Lam.) Taub. (Fabaceae)** *Dhauk, Palas, Tesu, Khankra*

Erect tree, young stem clothed with grey or brown silky hairs; leaves alternate, petioles 7.5-15.0 cm long, trifoliate, leaflets 10 - 20 cm long, leathery, lower surface covered with dense silky hairs; racemes 15 cm long; flowers thickly clothed on the outside with silvery small hairs; pods narrowed suddenly into a stalk longer than calyx. Common throughout the hilly tracts; rarely on blackish clayey soil of plains. Fl. & Fr.: March- June.

Gum of *Butea monosperma* is very effective for removal of external parasites. Flowers of *Butea monosperma* are mixed with fodder of the animal for disposal of placenta after delivery. In foot and mouth disease the feet of the animal are washed with boiled mixture of its urine and 200 gm bark powder of *Butea monoperma*. Warmed bark extract is given orally to animal suffering from gastroenteritis. The bark paste is applied on the fractured bone of domestic animals. The bark powder is mixed with the ash of *Capparis decidua* and given orally to treat fractured bones. 100 gm decoction of bark is given orally against snake bite.

Blumea lacera **(Burm. f.) DC. (Asteraceae)** *Phatakdi, Kakronda*

Aromatic herb; leaves obovate- oblong, viscid; head in spiciform leafy compound panicles. Common in wet and shady localities. Fl. & Fr.: February – June.

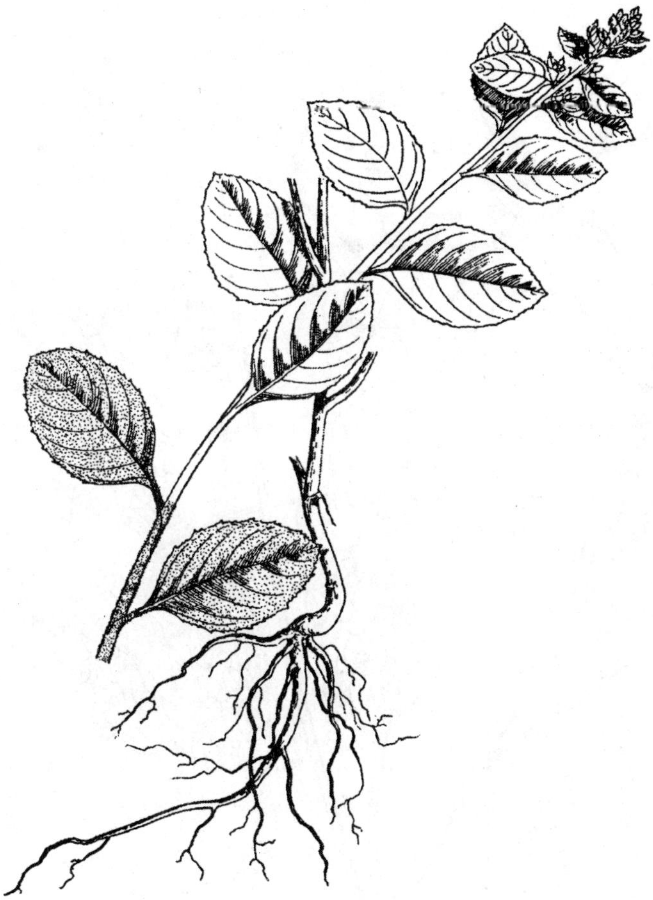

Fig. 25. *Blumea lacera* (Burm. f.) DC.

The paste of leaves is applied locally on wounds of animals to kill the worms.

Caesalpinia bonduc (Linn.) Roxb. (Caesalpiniaceae)
Kantkaranj, Katha (Plate 4)

An extensively climbing or scrambling shrub covered with short, straight prickles, those on the leaf rachis reflexes branchlets fulvous hairy; leaves simple or large persistent compound or pinnatifid, stipules foliaceous, pinna 6-8 pairs; flowers pale yellow; young pods softly echinate, old broad-oblong, prickly, dehiscent, 1 to 2 seeded. Grows in dry and semiarid regions, usually in open hedges; evergreen. Fl. & Fr.: August – April.

50 g seed powder is given orally to treat fever, worms and flatulence. 50 ml decoction of roots with the paste of 11 black peppers (*Piper nigrum*) is given to cows for disposal of retained placenta after delivery.

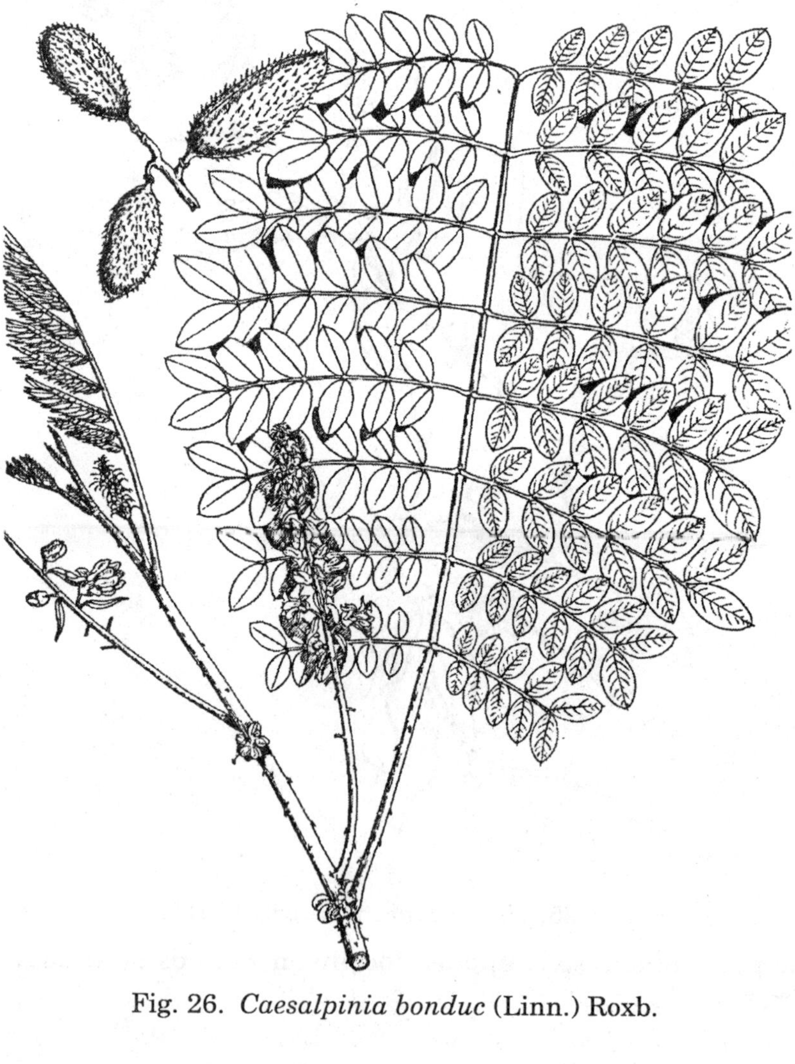

Fig. 26. *Caesalpinia bonduc* (Linn.) Roxb.

***Calligonum polygonoides* Linn. (Polygonaceae)** *Phog* (Plate 4)

Much branched, woody upto 2.5 m high shrub; leaves small, linear short-lived; flowers pinkish, fasciculate in the axils of ochreae; fruits oblong, clothed with reddish-brown bristles. A typical sand dune plant forms an association with *Leptadenia pyrotechnica* and *Aerva javanica.* Fl. & Fr.: March - June rarely in December.

Extract of the plant is given to treat constipation. Decoction of whole plant is given to treat urinary problems. The extract of plant is given to animals through drenching tube to treat colic whereas decoction of whole plant is given to treat dysuria.

***Calotropis gigantea* (Linn.) R.Br. (Asclepiadaceae)** *Safad Akdo*

Tree; leaves sessile or with petiole 0.2-0.7 mm long; inflorescence of 1-3 fascicles; flowers 14-15 mm by 3-4.5 cm diam.; pedicels 2.5-3.2 cm long, sepals lanceolate-ovate to ovate, 5-7 mm long, corolla subrotate; lobes ovate, 15-17 mm by 10-11 mm wide, cream-tipped internally, staminal corona lobes 11-12 mm by 6-6.5 mm wide, broadly flanged, cream, with base elongated into an upturned vesicle ca 5 mm long. Occurs widely in wastelands of arid regions. Fl. & Fr.: Most of the year.

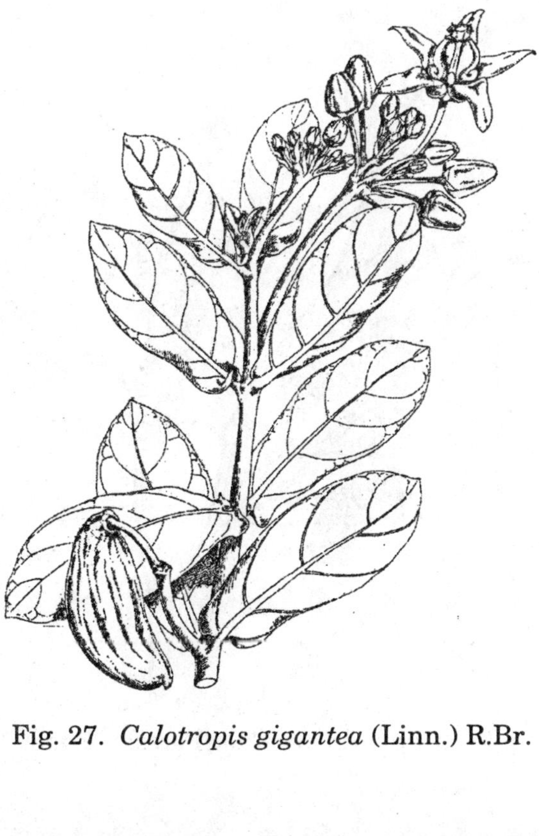

Fig. 27. *Calotropis gigantea* (Linn.) R.Br.

Poultice of roasted leaves is tied to treat swelling as well as on dislocated joints, sprains and fractured bone.

***Calotropis procera* Br. (Asclepiadaceae)** *Akdo, Aak, Aakro* (Plate 4)

A stout, hoary, tomentose shrub; leaves opposite, simple, oblong, cordate; peduncles often paired, tomentose and often branched; flowers about 12 mm, having lobes erect, white with purple blotch on the upper half, coronal process with a purple tinge, obtuse, muticous tip and fleshy upturned white base; follicles recurved, somewhat sausage-shaped, outer and inner coats with fibrous tissue between; seeds ovate, 6 mm, smooth with long comas. Occurs widely in wastelands of arid region. Fl. & Fr.: Most of the year.

Four to five drops of the fresh latex of the plant is dropped on the injured portion as an antiseptic. Mixture of 50 ml hydrochloric acid (HCl), 50 ml latex of *Calotropis procera* and 50 ml latex of *Mangifera indica* is prepared and used as an antidote to scorpion bite.

***Capparis decidua* (Forssk.) Edgew. (Capparaceae)** *Kair, Ker* (Plate 4)

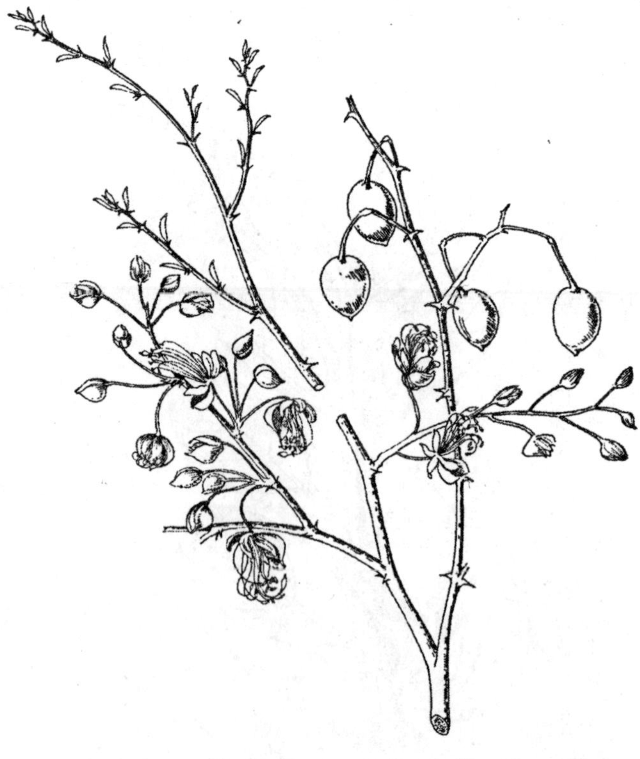

Fig. 28. *Capparis decidua* (Forssk.) Edgew.

Leafless, much branched, dense shrub, thorns in pairs, straight; glabrous, linear; pungent leaves found on very young shoots; flowers in simple corymbs on short lateral shoots, red brown, 2.5 cm in diameter; fruits 1.25-1.9 cm, glabrous, long - beaked. Commonly occur throughout the desert on hard gravelly and clayey soil, rarely on sandy plains and dunes. Fl. & Fr.: March-July.

Decoction of ½ kg shoots of *Cissus quadrangula*, ½ Kg ash of stem of *Capparis decidua* and ash of roots of *Ziziphus jujuba*, ½ Kg jaggery with milk is given to the animal once in a day, till the healing of fractured bone.

***Capparis sepiaria* Linn. (Capparaceae)** *Katar, Kali- Katar*

A large climbing shrub, thorns curved; leaves elliptic; petioles 0.2 cm long; umbels simple; flowers white, pedicles short; fruit borne in clusters, pisiform, black. Preferably grows in dry climate. Fl. & Fr.: March – August.

Oil of *Ricinus communis,* crushed rhizomes of *Curcuma longa* and jaggery are mixed in equal ratio i.e. 2 kg each. 250 g of this mixture is mixed with 250 g coal prepared from wood of *Capparis sepiaria* and given to the animal with 1 kg of milk. This heals up the fractured bone fast if given daily. Extract of root is given orally to animals in diphtheria.

***Capsicum annum* Linn. (Solanaceae)** *Lal-mirch*

Perennial herb; leaves lanceolate; white flowers and slender, green, red or orange berries; calyx enclosing the base of berry. Cultivated throughout the area for its edible berries. Fl. & Fr.: Throughout the year.

Paste of dried fruit powder is mixed with sugar and applied in the throat of animal to treat tonsillitis.

***Capsicum minimum* Roxb. (Solanaceae)** *Rukunimirshi*

Perennial herbs; with lanceolate leaves; flowers white and slender; green, red or orange fruits. Fl. & Fr.: September – December.

Paste of ripe fruits is fed to animal 4 to 5 times in a day to treat stomach disorder.

Cardiospermum halicacabum Linn. (**Sapindaceae**) *Chirphut, Parpotiea, Kanfuti*

Annual wiry herb; thinly pubescent or nearly glabrous with acuminate leaflets; flowers white, very minute; capsules depressed, pyriform; seeds tomentose, globose. Mainly in wastelands; plains to the lower slopes. Fl. & Fr.: July - March

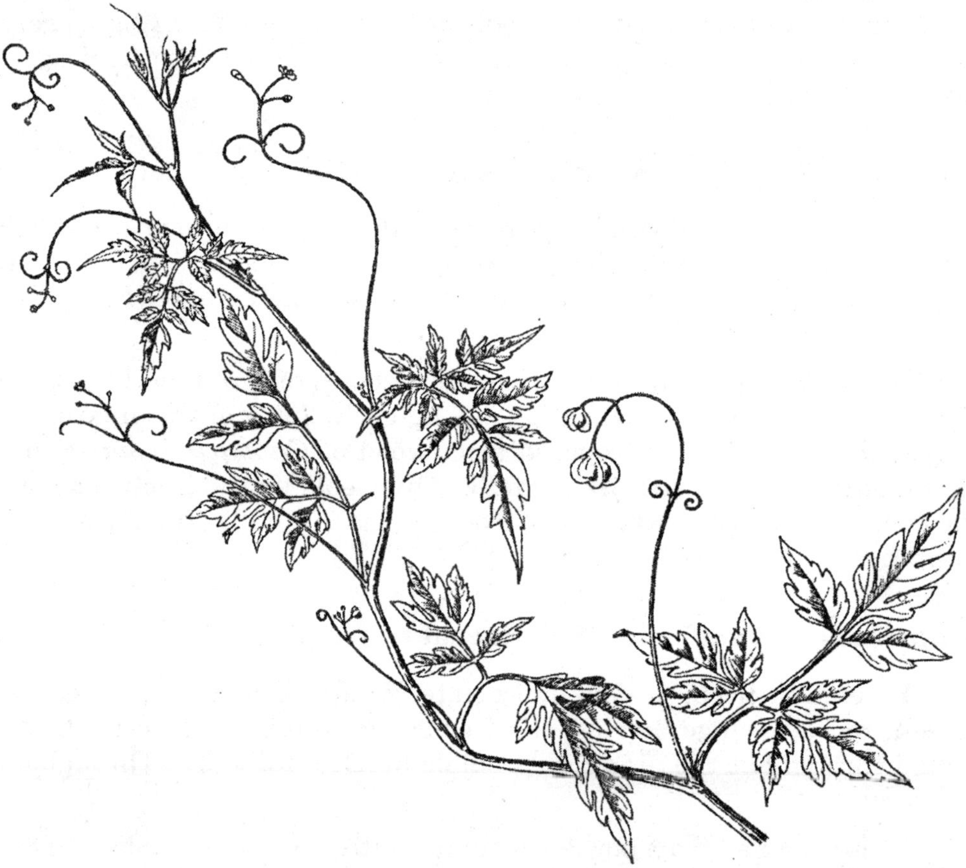

Fig. 29. *Cardiospermum halicacabum* Linn.

Leaf paste is applied on the body to kill lice and other parasitic insects.

***Carica papaya* Linn. (Caricaceae)** *Papita, Hajarkakri*

Soft wooded, dioecious tree with usually unbranched trunk and milky sap; leaves in terminal cluster, palmately lobed; fruit a berry; laticiferous glands occurs in roots, stem, leaves and fruits. The plant thrives best in rich soil of uniform texture. Fl. & Fr.: Throughout the year.

Latex of *Carica papaya* is applied on the skin to treat eczema.

***Carissa congesta* Wt. (Apocynaceae)** *Karonda*

Erect or scandent shrubs, armed with straight, paired horizontal spines; leaves 2-6 by 1.5-4.0 cm, elliptic-oblong to ovate, acute, mucronate; flowers white, in corymbose cymes. Usually met with in the forests and wastelands. Fl. & Fr.: January – April

Latex of *Carissa congesta* is applied on the fractured bone or dislocated joint for early healing.

***Cassia angustifolia* Vahl (Caesalpiniaceae)** *Sonamukhi*

Shrub; leaves usually 5-8 jugate, leaflets oval, lanceolate, glabrous; racemes axillary erect, waxy many-flowered, usually considerably exceeding the subtending leaf; bracts membranous, ovate or obovate, caduceous; pods are 3.5-7 cm by 2 cm wide, greenish brown to dark brown in colour and contain 5-7 obovate dark brown and nearly smooth seeds. Cultivated plant. Fl. & Fr.: August – December.

Leaves are fed to the camel to treat flatulence.

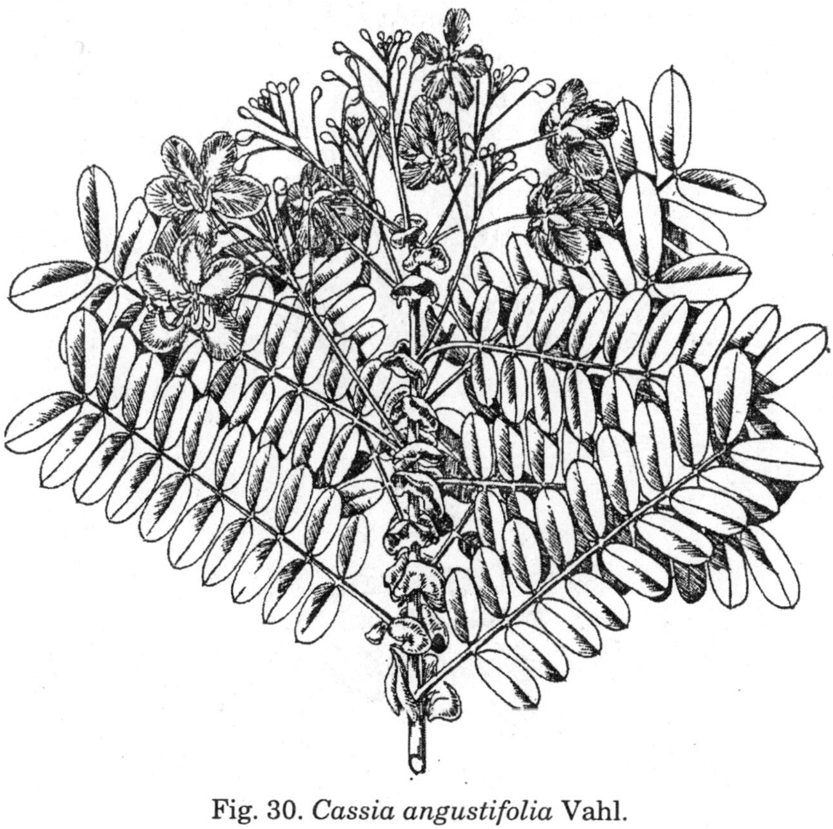

Fig. 30. *Cassia angustifolia* Vahl.

***Cassia auriculata* Linn. (Caesalpiniaceae)** *Anwal, Tarwan*

A much branched handsome shrub, 1.0-3.25 m high with hairy twigs; leaves pinnately compound, leaflets 8-12 pairs; flowers large, yellow in subterminal corymbs; pods 0.75-1.25 cm by 1.75 cm, flat, obtuse at each end; seeds 6-10. Xerophytic in nature; wild in dry regions, cultivated in other areas; prefers cottony soils. Fl. & Fr.: October – March.

Tender shoots of plant grinded with buttermilk and jaggery is given orally to treat dysentery. Leaf paste is applied locally to treat boils, swellings and wounds.

***Cassia tora* Linn. (Caesalpiniaceae)** *Punwad, Punwadia*

A small weed, subshrub, upto 75-150 cm; branchlets glabrous; leaves upto 4 cm long, leaflet 3 pairs, obovate, thin, coriaceous, glabrous above, pubescent below; racemes terminal, corymbose; pods short, stipitate, flat, compressed; seeds oblong, longitudinal. Sparsely distributed from plains to the hills; often found in association with *Cassia obtusifolia*. Fl. & Fr.: August – November.

Boiled seeds are given to the animals to treat hypogalactia.

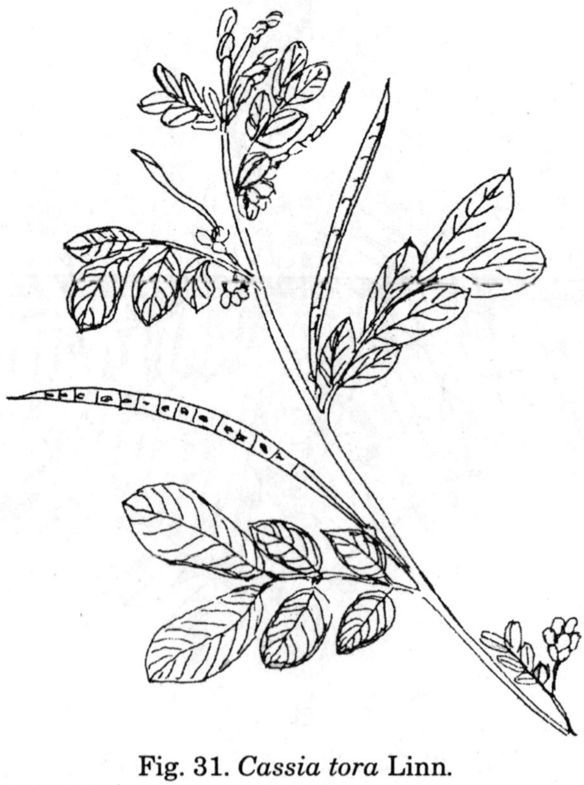

Fig. 31. *Cassia tora* Linn.

Cassia fistula **Linn. (Caesalpiniaceae)** *Amaltas, Bahawa, Garmale, Karmalo*

A tree with grey bark; pinnate leaves; flowers yellow, blossoms in pendant racemes; fruits elongated, brown to black, cylindrical lomentum with numerous compartments. Prefers laterite soil; often planted as road side tree. Fl. & Fr.: May- June.

Two-three pods are fed to the animal to treat flatulence. Decoction of about 100 g of pods or stem bark (if pods are not available) of *Cassia fistula* is given to the animal as a purgative.

Catunaregam spinosa **(Thunb.) Tiruv. (Rubiaceae)** *Kharedi*

A large deciduous armed shrub upto 9 m in height with strong spines; leaves simple, wrinkled; flowers at first white, later turning yellow, fragrant, solitary or 2-3 together at the ends of short leaf bearing branchlets; fruits globose berries yellow when ripe, crowned with large calyx limb; seeds many angular, embedded in the pulp. Sparsely distributed from plains to the hills. Fl. & Fr.: March – June.

About 500 g of whole plant, 50 g of jaggery and 25 g of dried rhizome powder of *Curcuma longa* is given to animal with fodder to treat diarrhoea.

Celastrus paniculata **Willd. (Celastraceae)** *Mal - kangni, Mali* (Plate 4)

Large climbing shrub, unarmed straggler/liane upto 12 m, branchlets puberulose; leaves alternate, ovate to orbicular, thin, coriaceous, base obtuse to subacute, margin dentate, petiole upto 3 cm; panicle terminal; flowers polygamous, greenish white; capsules 0.6-1.0 cm; seeds 6, ellipsoid to ovoid, upto 5 mm. Extensive straggler as liane on trees; common in dry deciduous forests, particularly in the east of Aravalli. Fl. & Fr.: March – September.

One cup infusion of seeds is given orally to the animal for seven days to treat paralysis. Seed oil mixed with seed oil of *Sesamum indicum* is massaged to treat paralysis.

Celosia argentea **Linn. (Amaranthaceae)** *Surli, Garkha* (Plate 4)

Common weed; herb upto 1-2 m; leaves elliptic-ovate below, linear-lanceolate above; spikes dense, cylindric, very showy; flowers 4 mm across, pink, gradually turning white, bract lanceolate 6 mm, scarious; capsules globose, reticulate. On hills in arable lands, as a weed of cultivated field; conspicuous in harvested field; less common in plains. Fl. & Fr.: August- November.

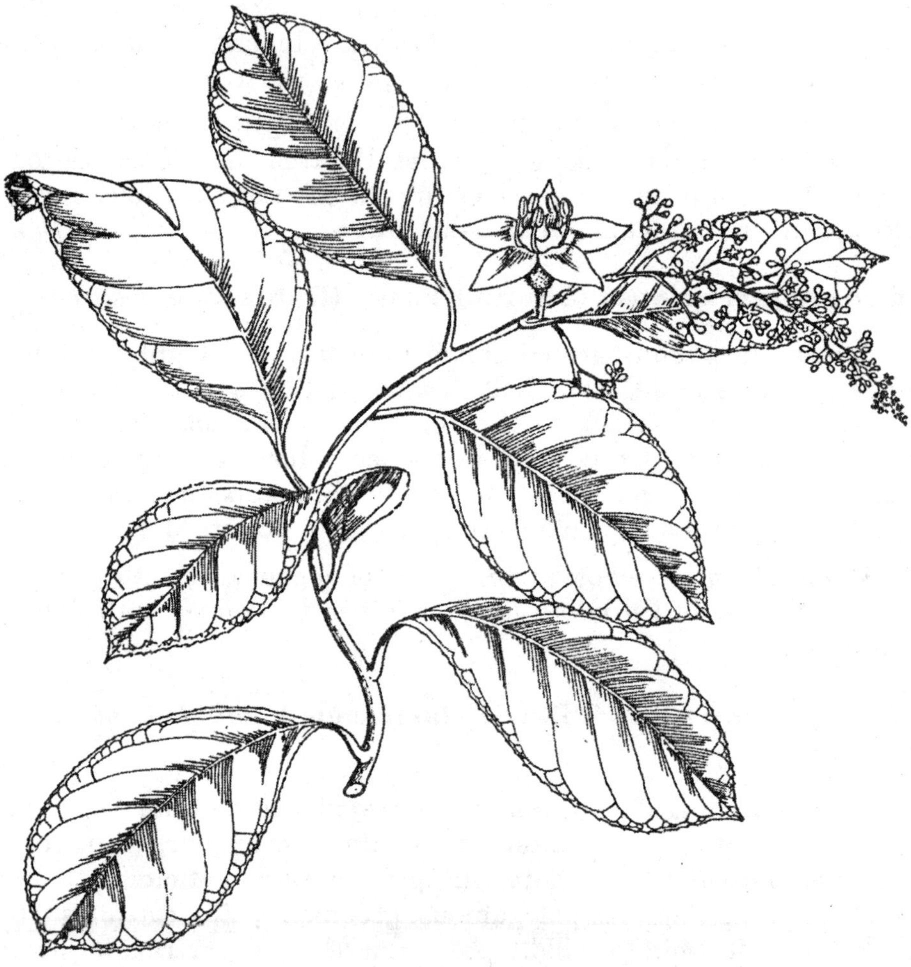

Fig. 32. *Celastrus paniculata* Willd.

Root extract of *Celosia argentea* mixed with *Tamarindus indica* fruits or leaves is given orally to treat food-poisoning.

Ceropegia attenuata **Hook. (Asclepiadaceae)** *Khadula*

Tall, tuberous herb; leaves subsessile, linear, acute, tapering at base; cymes axillary or extra axillary, shortly peduncled, 1 to 2 flowered. Rare, in exposed rocky grounds. Fl. & Fr.: July – October.

Bulbs and leaves are given to animal orally to remove the stone in urinary tract.

***Ceropegia bulbosa* Roxb. (Asclepiadaceae)** *Khadula* (Plate 4)

Twining, perennial herb, with an underground, tuberous stem; leaves glabrous; cymes pedunculate, 6 to 10 flowered; seeds linear - oblong with membranous wings. Rare, in exposed rocky habitats, particularly on hillocks. Fl. & Fr.: July-December.

Leaves of *Ceropegia bulbosa* are given as fodder as a prophylactic measure against tumour formation.

***Chenopodium album* Linn. (Chenopodiaceae)**
Bathua, Chilario, Kaligera

Herb; leaves oblong rhomboid; flowers born in clusters in paniculate, ebracteate spikes; seeds rugose. Weed in cultivated fields, gardens and other humid places. Fl. & Fr.: October – April.

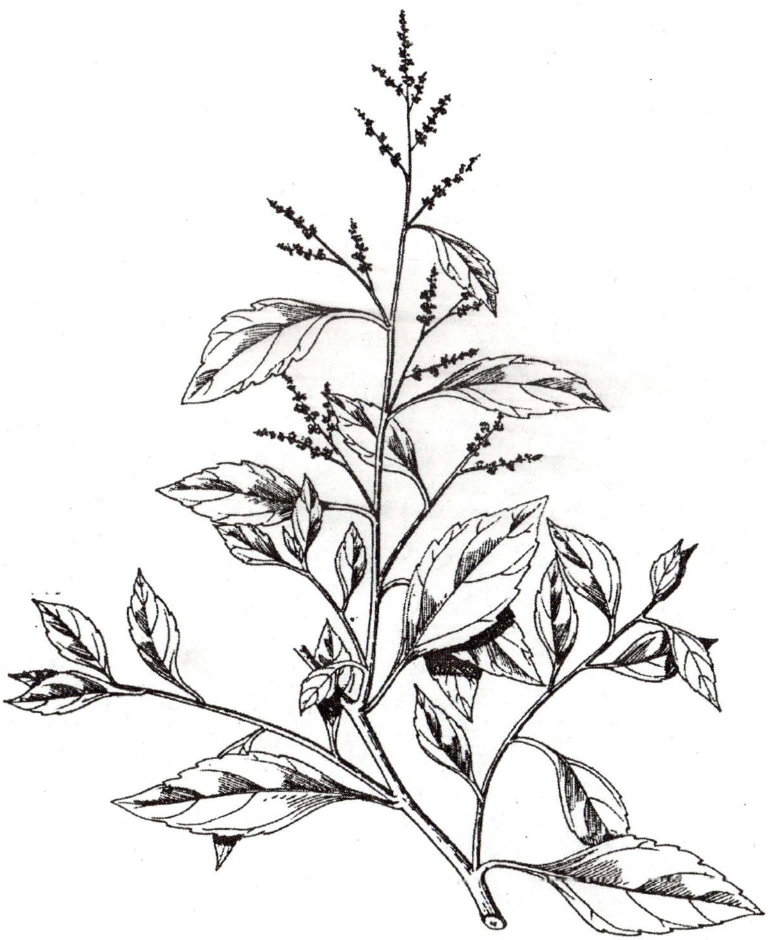

Fig. 33. *Chenopodium album* Linn.

Paste made from leaves is applied on wounds of animals for early healing.

Chlorophytum tuberosum **(Roxb.) Baker (Liliaceae)**
Safed musli, Futra (Plate 4)

Annual herb, with small root stock and many cylindric root fibres ending in ellipsoid tubers; leaves linear-lanceolate, acute, undulate, margined; scape solitary, scattered flowers forming dense racemes; seeds irregularly orbicular usually compressed, pitted, black. Rare, on the hills of protected areas. Fl. & Fr.: June- October.

Three to four tubers of *Chlorophytum tuberosum* are mixed with fodder of animal to treat diarrhoea. It also acts as a galactgogue.

Cicer arietinum **Linn. (Fabaceae)** *Chana*

Much–branched herbs, with pinnate leaves and turgid-oblong fruits. Commonly cultivated as a winter season crop. Fl. & Fr.: December – March.

Fresh leaf extract is given to animal to treat constipation.

Cissampelos pareira **Linn. (Menispermaceae)** *Kalipar* (Plate 4)

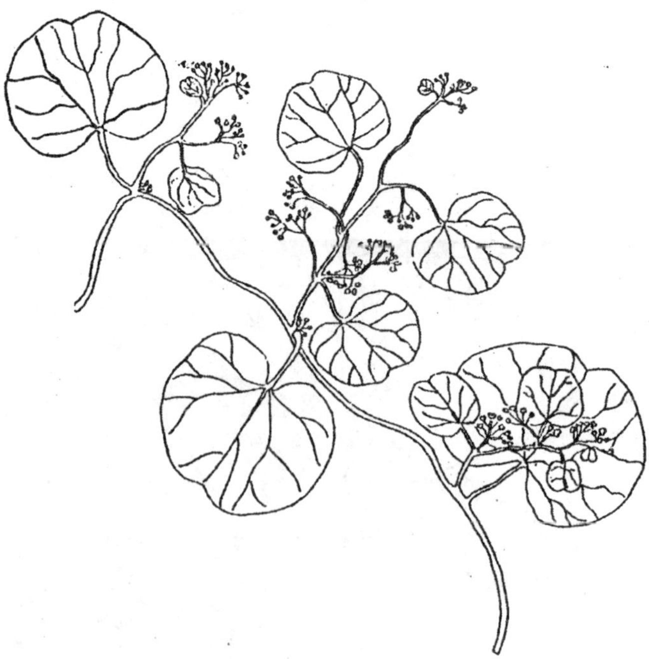

Fig. 34. *Cissampelos pareira* Linn.

Twining perennial shrub; leaves reniform, orbicular or cordate, 4.5 by 6.5 cm, peltate, chartaceous, 5 by 7 nerved, pubescent, base cordate or truncate; male inflorescence pendent type, flowers greenish; female inflorescence in thyroid clusters; fruits red when ripe, subtended by the conspicuous auricular bracts. More abundant on the degraded slopes; extensive tomentose climber as compact mats on thickets. Fl. & Fr.: July- October.

Extract of root is given to animal to treat snake-bite and dog bite as an antidote.

***Cissus quadrangula* Linn. (Vitaceae)** *Hadjore* (Plate 5)

A succulent twiner, rambling shrub, stem 4 angular, glabrous, winged or margined, contracted at the nodes; leaves simple, caducous; cymes umbellate; flowers 7 cm across, greenish yellow, red-tipped; berry globose, apiculate; seed smooth. In scrub jungles and wetlands upto 500 m on thickets. Fl. & Fr.: Throughout the year.

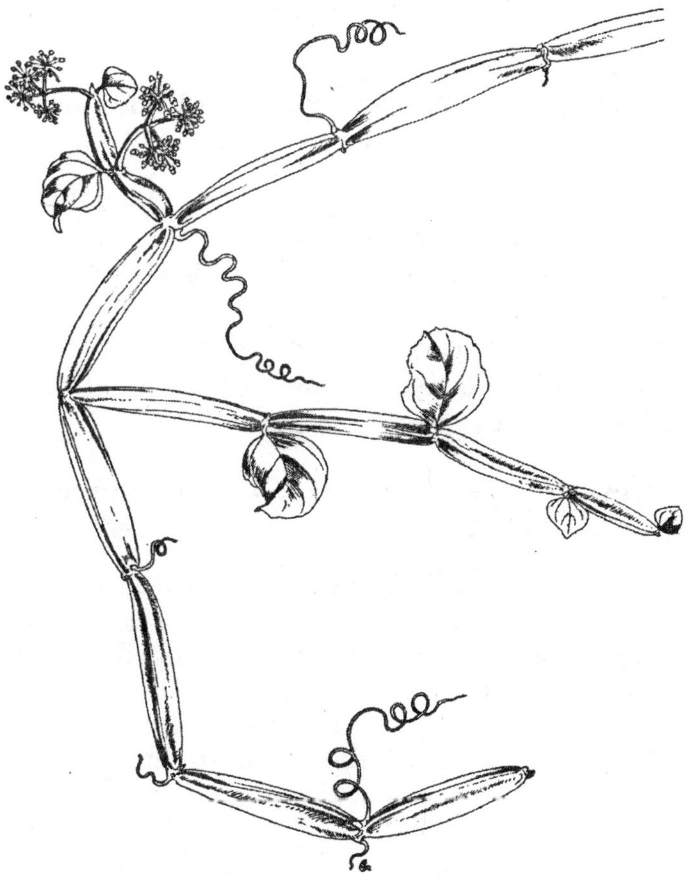

Fig. 35. *Cissus quandrangula* Linn.

Whole plant of *Cissus quadrangula* (200 g) is grinded with 50 g bark of *Wrightia tinctoria*, 50 g leaves of *Vitex negundo,* 50 g powder of *Piper nigrum* seeds and 50 g *Allium sativum* bulbs and given to the animal to treat foot and mouth disease. Paste of about three nodes is given to the animal with water through drenching tube once in a day for 8 to 10 days for early healing of fractured bone. Paste of stem is applied locally to treat sprain and swelling.

Cissus repanda **Vahl (Vitaceae)** *Panivala*

Large, woody climber with fissured, corky bark and vinaceous-purple stem and branches; tendrils with flattened disc; leaves pubescent above, silky tomentose beneath; flowers in umbel- like clusters, pedicelled pink; berries tipped by mucronate style, 1- seeded. Occasional, in deciduous forests, particularly in the east of Aravalli. Fl. & Fr.: May- August.

Root powder acts as lactgogue and is given to animal with fodder to increase milk secretion. Infusion of the climber is given orally to treat boils.

Cistanche tubulosa **(Schremk) Wight. (Orobanchaceae)**
Lauki-mula

Purplish-yellow, leafless root-parasites, having solitary or fascicled from the ground, upto 60 cm high; scapes furrowed, fleshy, pubescent, terminating into 2-4 cm long spikes; capsules 20-25 by 8-10 mm, ovoid-oblong, laterally compressed, beaked by seeds numerous, reticulately pitted. Fl. & Fr.: October-March.

Paste of whole plant is applied for the treatment of Bovine viral mammaitis (BVM). It acts as anti-allergic.

Citrullus colocynthis **(Linn.) Schard. (Cucurbitaceae)**
Gartumba, Tumba (Plate 5)

Perennial trailing herb, branchlets hirsute; leaves alternate, simple, petiolate, ovate or narrowly triangular, deeply trilobed, lobes pinnatifid, triangular, chartaceous, rigid; tendril simple, slender, petiole upto 3 cm; male flower 1 cm across, yellow; in female flower, ovary ovoid; fruit globose, striped green and white when young, yellow when ripe. Common in sandy habitats, particularly in the desertic zones. Fl. & Fr.: Almost throughout the year.

Decoction of fruits is given to the animal twice a day to treat constipation. A mixture of 20 g honey, 20 g extract of roots of *Citrullus colocynthis*, 20 g mustard oil is applied internally to reduce the pain during delivery. Pulp of roasted fruits mixed with flour of *Pennisetum typhoides* and salt is fed to the animal to treat impaction with fever. Roasted fruits and decoction of roots is given to the domestic animal to treat constipation, digestive disorders and gastritis.

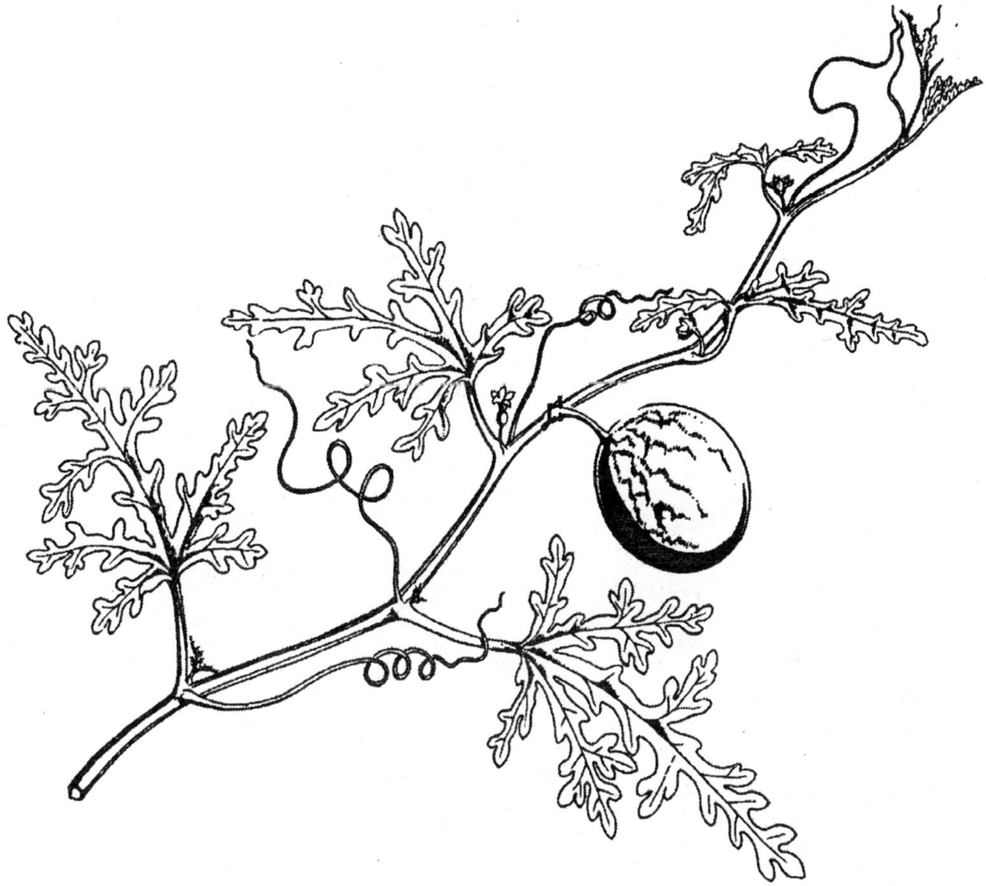

Fig. 36. *Citrullus colocynthis* (Linn.) Schard.

***Citrus medica* Linn. (Rutaceae)** *Bijora* (Plate 5)

An evergreen armed shrub with straggling thorny branches and smooth yellowish brown bark; leaves oblong or elliptic, coriaceous, pullucid-punctate; flower in axillary cymes; fruit large berries, oblong or globose, fleshy, rind thick, rough, irregular or warted. Commonly cultivated for its fruits. Fl. & Fr.: Summer and winter.

Fruit powder is given to the animal to dissolve the iron piece engulfed by the animal accidentally. Juice of 10 lemons is given with 750g sugar to induce lactation.

Cleome gynandra **Linn. (Cleomaceae)** *Karelia, Safed- bagra*

Glandular hairy herbs; leaves 3- to 5 foliolate; flowers in terminal racemes; capsules linear- cylindric. Common weed in wastelands during rainy season. Fl. & Fr.: July-December.

Paste of leaves of *Cleome gynandra* is applied locally twice a day to treat eczema.

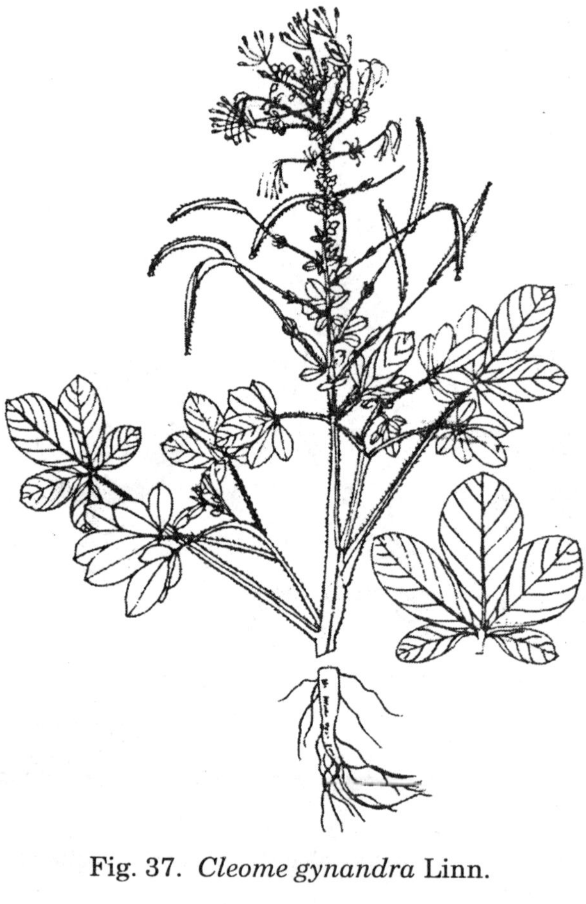

Fig. 37. *Cleome gynandra* Linn.

Cleome viscosa **Linn. (Cleomaceae)** *Singali, Bagra*

Pubescent, annual, woody at base; 3- to 5- foliolate leaves; flowers in leafy racemes; capsule cylindric, beaked. Common in cultivated fields during rainy season. Fl. & Fr.: July - November

Paste of about 50 g seeds of *Cleome viscosa* is given with water through drenching tube, thrice a day to treat diarrhoea and fever.

Paste is prepared by mixing equal amount of leaves of this plant with leaves of *Azadirachta indica,* and applied externally on the skin of animal for killing ectoparasites *e.g.* lices and ticks. Decoction of mixture of roots and leaves is used to give water bath to animal to treat body swelling and bodyache.

Extract prepared from the flowers of *Madhuca indica* and *Clerodendrum viscosum* is given orally to the animal early in the morning for 15 days to 3 months to treat arthritis and rheumatism.

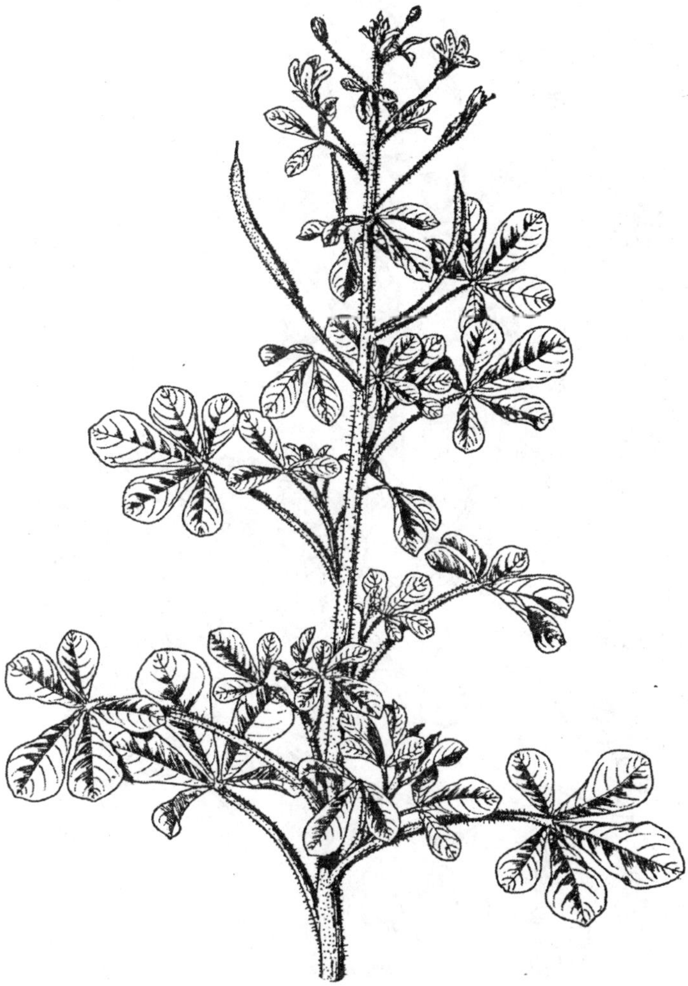

Fig. 38. *Cleome viscosa* Linn.

***Clerodendrum phlomidis* L.f. (Verbenaceae)** *Arni, Anni*

Shrub, 1-3 m tall; stem and branches whitish pubescent; leaves petiolate, rhomboid-ovate, flowers fragrant, in axillary and terminal panicles; fruit drupes 0.5-1.25 cm long with persistent calyx. Common throughout the plains. Fl. & Fr.: August – March.

Paste prepared by mixing equal amount of leaves of this plant with leaves of *Azadirachta indica* is applied externally on the skin of animal for killing ectoparasites *e.g.* lices and ticks. Decoction of mixture of roots and leaves is used to give bath to animal to treat body swelling and bodyache.

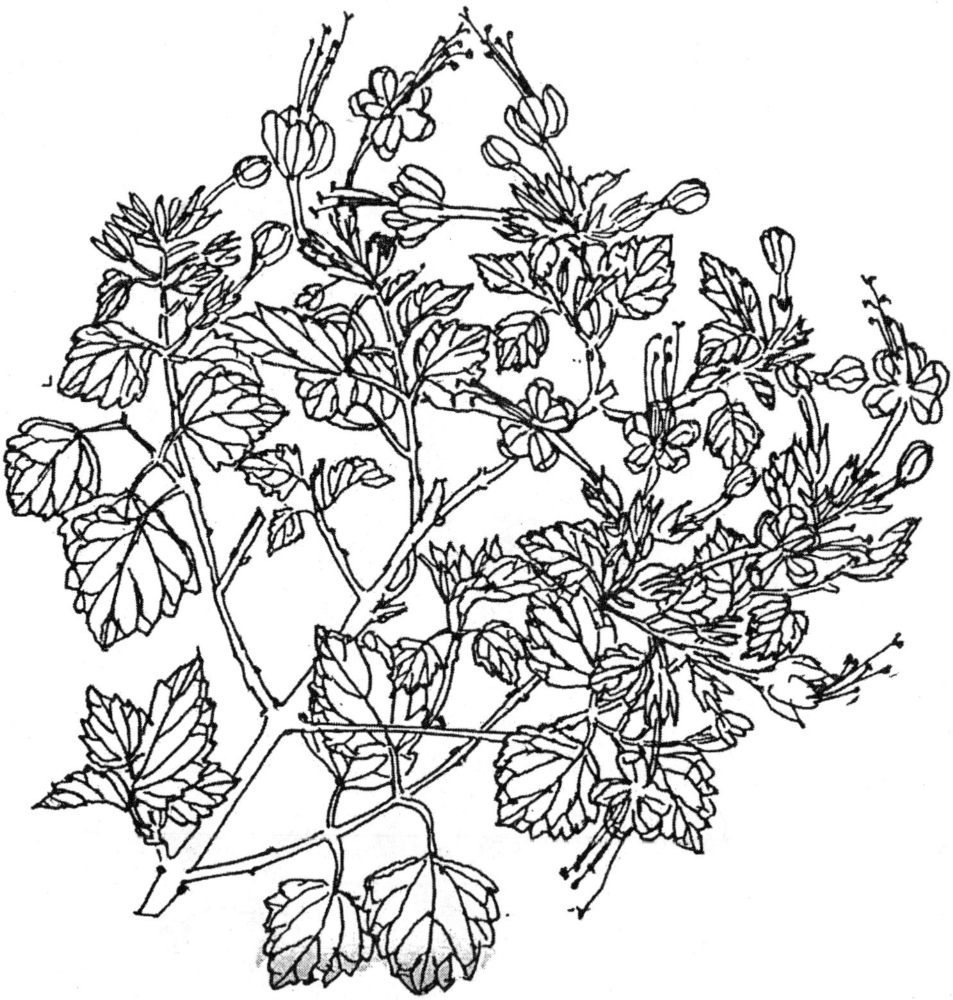

Fig. 39. *Clerodendrum phlomidis* L.f.

***Clitoria ternatea* Linn. (Fabaceae)** *Gokarni* (Plate 5)

Handsome twining perennial herb with terete stem and branches; leaves compound, imparipinnate, flowers solitary, axillary or in fascicles; pods sharply beaked; seeds reniform. Common garden plant; occurs in hedges all over the tropical regions. Fl. & Fr.: Most part of the year.

Seeds of *Clitoria ternatea* are given with jaggery or chapatti to treat constipation. Dose depends on body weight of the animal.

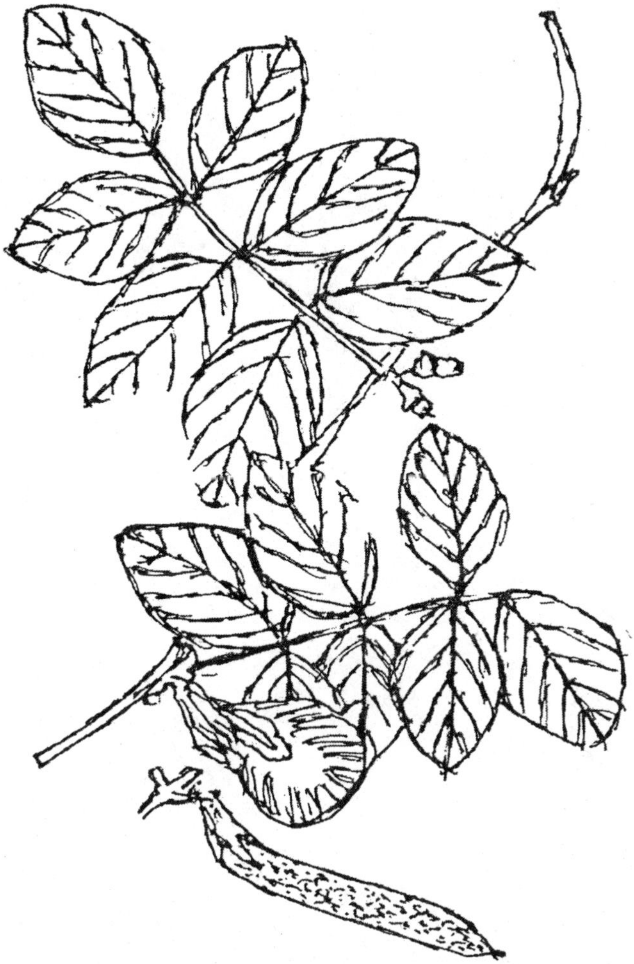

Fig. 40. *Clitoria ternatea* Linn.

***Coccinia grandis* (Linn.) J.O. Voigt (Cucurbitaceae)** *Tindori*

Perennial, much branched, handsome tendril climber; roots tuberous; leaves deltoid or subrotund, palmately 5-nerved; flowers unisexual; fruits ovoid or oblong or ellipsoid berries. Semi wild; common in thickets and wastelands. Fl. & Fr.: Throughout the year.

Leaves are grinded with *Piper betel* and paste is rubbed on the body to treat allergy. Extract of the leaves grinded with ghee is dropped into nostrils to treat epistaxis. Extract of leaves is dropped in eyes to treat opacity of cornea.

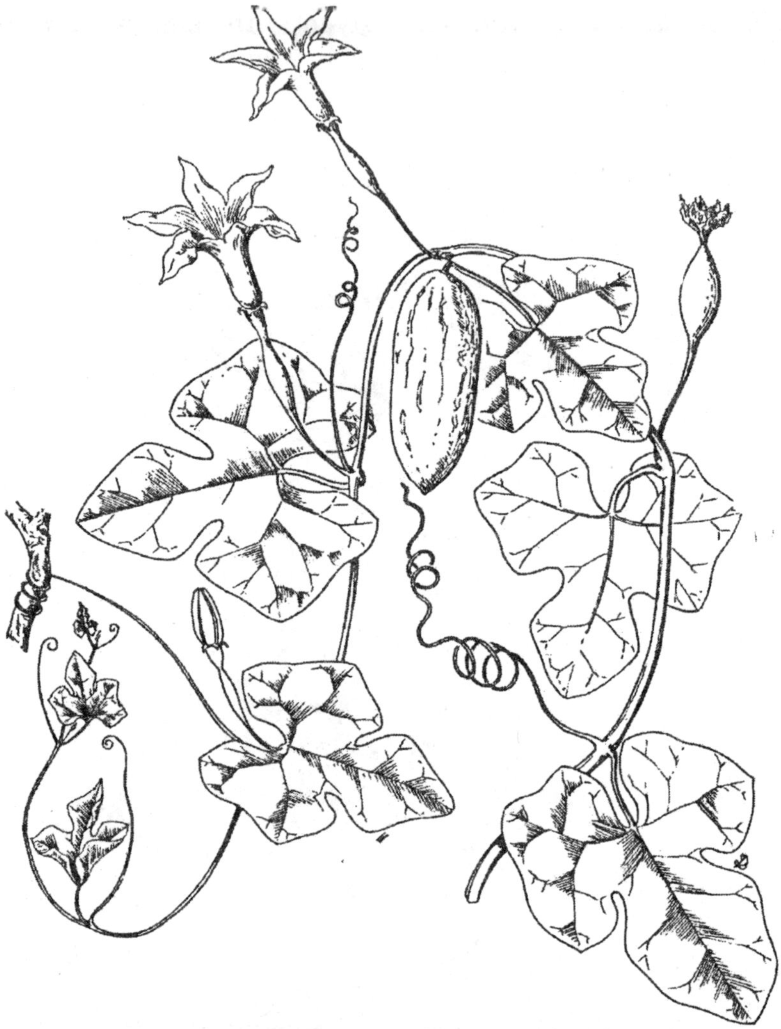

Fig. 41. *Coccinia grandis* (Linn.) J.O. Voigt

Cocculus hirsutus (Linn.) Diels (Menispermaceae) *Bajar- bel, Van- veela, Baar* (Plate 5)

Scandent herb; bark, corky, young parts densely hairy; leaves petiolate; lamina base cordate to cuneate, surface pubescent. Restricted to hilly tracts, usually occurs in association with *Euphorbia neriifolia* and *Lycium barbarum*. Fl. & Fr.: Almost round the year.

Leaves (10 g) of *Cocculus hirsutus* are fed to the animal once in a day for three days to treat dog-bite. Leaf extract is rubbed on the body and after one hour, bath is given to the animal for complete removal of external parasites.

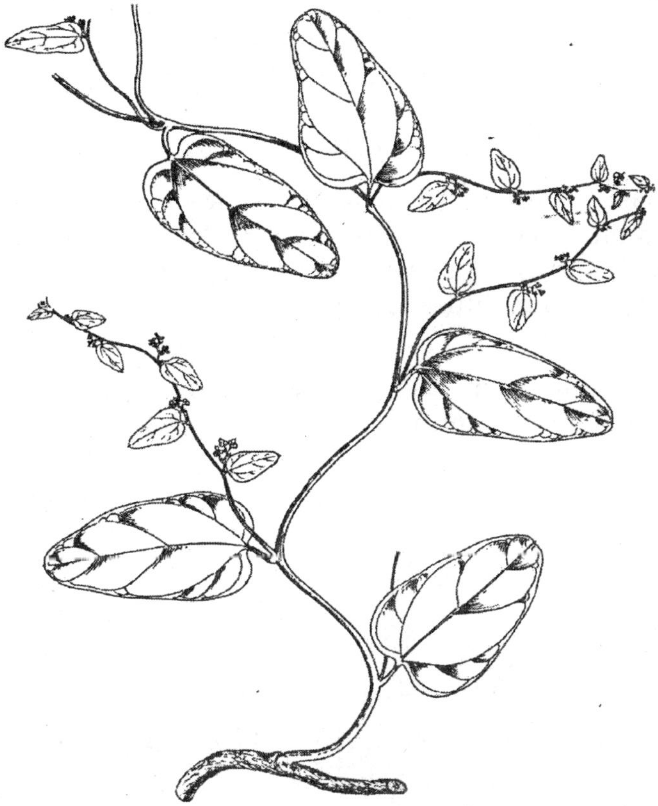

Fig. 42. *Cocculus hirsutus* (Linn.) Diels

Cocculus pendulus (J.R. & G. Forst.) Diels (Menispermaceae)
Pilwani, Khangro

Twiner; bark blackish-brown; leaves petiolate, 1 cm long; lamina base cuneate to cordate, ovate-oblong to ovate-lanceolate, 1-9 by 0.2-4.5 cm, emarginate to mucronulate at apex. Common on sandy plains. Fl. & Fr.: October- December.

Mixture of 100 g wood ash of this plant and 100 g cow's milk fat is given to the animal to treat mastitis.

Commelina forsskalaei Vahl. (Commelinaceae) *Mirja*

Much-branched, diffuse, annual herbs; leaves linear or narrowly oblong-elliptic, often undulate; cymes axillary, branched, 3 to 5-flowered; cleistogamous flowers usually solitary in a spathe, bisexual, reduced, with usually 1-seeded capsule. Common in cultivated fields, in marshy places and often in the forests. Fl. & Fr.: August-November.

About 250 ml extract of whole plant is given to the animal twice in a day for 15 days to treat rheumatism and body swelling. The extract also massaged for the same.

***Commiphora wightii* (Arn.) Bhandari (Burseraceae)** *Gugal*

Handsome deciduous tree with papery bark and greenish soft wood; leaves alternate, imparipinnate, leaflets opposite; flowers small in fascicles; fruits ovoid or subglobose, fleshy drupes as big as pea. Rare, on the open dry hills and other rocky habitats. Fl. & Fr.: February – June.

Chopped stem and leaves mixed with buttermilk is kept in earthen pot and given to animal to treat rheumatism.

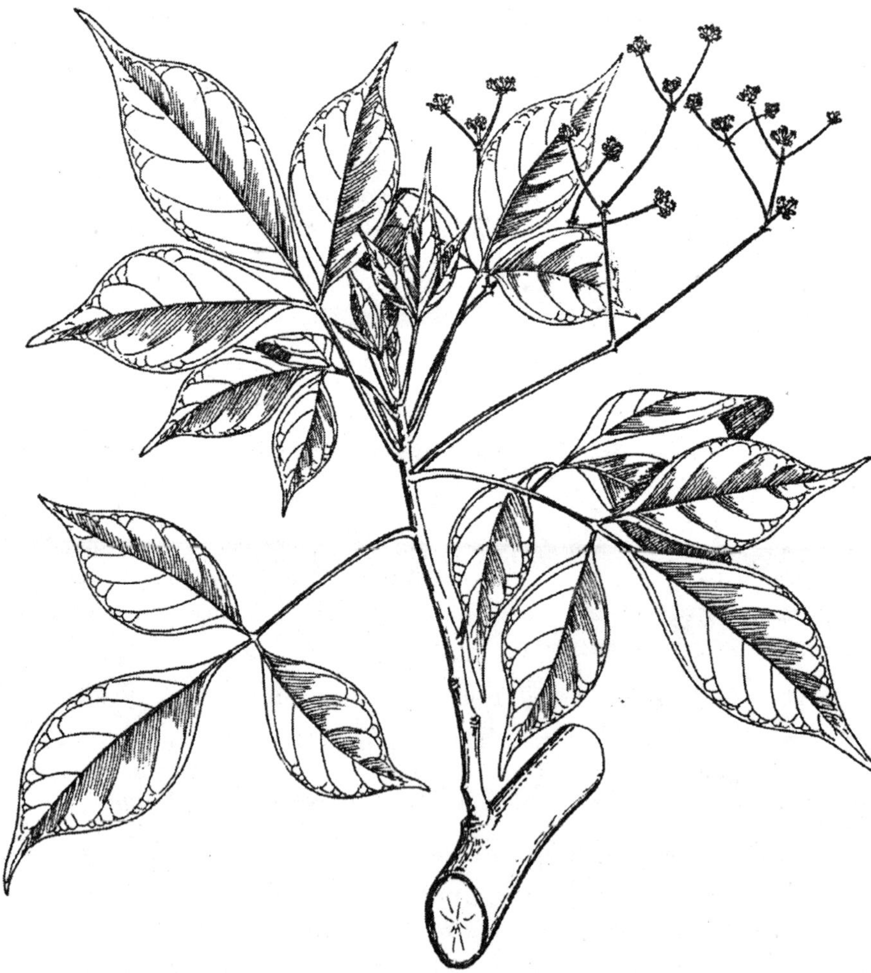

Fig. 43. *Commiphora wightii* (Arm.) Bhandari

***Corallocarpus epigaeus* (Rottl. & Willd.) Hook. f. (Cucurbitaceae)** *Marsiakand, Kadwi- nai, Mirch bel, Kadvi bel* (Plate 5)

Perennial, climbing herb; roots napiform; stems slender, glabrous, angular-sulcate; leaves variable in size and shape, broadly suborbicular; tendrils simple, subfiliform, glabrous; fruits ovoid, base attenuate, red, 5 to 8 seeded. Found in sandy to gravelly habitats; not common. Fl. & Fr.: August – November.

About 250 g of paste prepared from one tuber of *Corallocarpus epigaeus* and whole plant of *Tinospora cordifolia* is fed to the animal twice in a day for 3 days to treat tonsillitis.

***Corchorus depressus* (Linn.) Stocks. (Tiliaceae)** *Baphuli, Kagler, Chamaks*

Prostrate, much branched, woody perennial; leaves upto 2.5-1.2 cm, elliptic, crenate - serrate, plicate in bud; flowers in leaf-opposed cymes; capsules oblong-cylindric; beak short, straight or curved. Common in open gravelly places, abundant particularly in desert zone. Fl. & Fr.: August – March.

Leaves are fed to camel to treat stomachache. Whole plant crushed with water is given to animal to increase the secretion of milk.

***Cordia dichotoma* Forst. f. (Ehretiaceae)** *Lasora, Gunda, Lesuwa*

Medium- sized tree with a short trunk; leaves simple, elliptic-lanceolate; flowers small in lax terminal or axillary cymes; fruits drupe. In warmer regions; wild and cultivated. Fl. & Fr.: February – June.

Paste of leaves of *Cordia dichotoma* is given to the animal with water to treat diarrhoea. Leaves and fruits of *Cordia dichotoma* are given as a fodder to the animal to treat leucorrhoea. Extract of *Cordia dichotoma* leaves is mixed with honey and applied on the mouth of the animal to treat swelling of foot and mouth disease.

***Coriandrum sativum* Linn. (Apiaceae)** *Dhania*

Glabrous, annual herb; flowers pale to bright rose or nearly white; fruits subglobose, prominently ribbed. Cultivated as a winter season crop. Fl. & Fr.: Throughout the year.

Powder of about 100 g fruits is given with sugar to female animal after mating for 3-4 times in a day to avoid vomiting of conception.

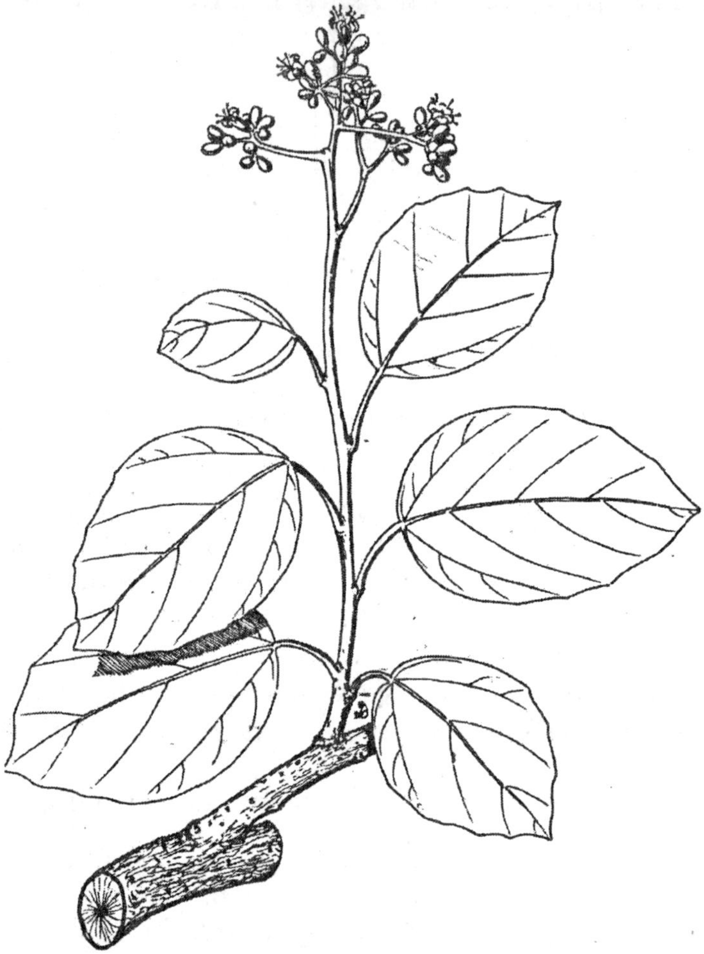

Fig. 44. *Cordia dichotoma* Forst. f.

Cosmostigma racemosa **(Roxb.) Wt. (Asclepiadaceae)** *Raidodi*

A shrubby twiner; leaves deciduous, ovate, acute, acuminate, glabrous, base cordate; flowers in axillary or sublateral cyme; follicles ovoid-oblong, bluntly pointed, smooth. Endemic to India. Fl. & Fr.: June - August.

Powder of pods is mixed with curd and given orally twice in a day to sheep and goat to treat gastroenteritis.

Costus speciosus **(Koen.) Sm. (Costaceae)** *Mahalakri* (Plate 6)

Succulent perennial herb with long leafy spirally twisted stems; 2-3 m high and horizontal rhizomes; leaves simple, spirally arranged, oblanceolate or oblong, glabrous above, silky pubescent beneath with broad leaf sheaths; flowers white large, scented, in large terminal spikes, bracts bright red; fruits globose/ovoid capsules; seeds obovoid or semiglobose. Rare, in dense protected forest of Southern Aravalli hills. Fl. & Fr.: August – December.

Pieces of rhizome are fed to the animals to treat rheumatism.

***Crinum asiaticum* Linn. (Amaryllidaceae)** *Jahari kanda*

A bulbous herb; bulb with a fusiform stoloniferous base, neck cylindric; leaves erect, 60 - 100 by 1.8 - 2.5 cm, linear, concave; scapes 45- 60 cm long, stout, umbels 6 to 15-flowered. Plant of swampy river bank; wild. Fl. & Fr.: Mainly in winter.

Tuber paste of *Crinum asiaticum* is applied on the skin for treatment of carbuncles. Extract of bulb mixed with curd is given orally to animal to treat flatulence. The poultice of tuber is tied to treat various skin diseases like abscesses, warts etc.

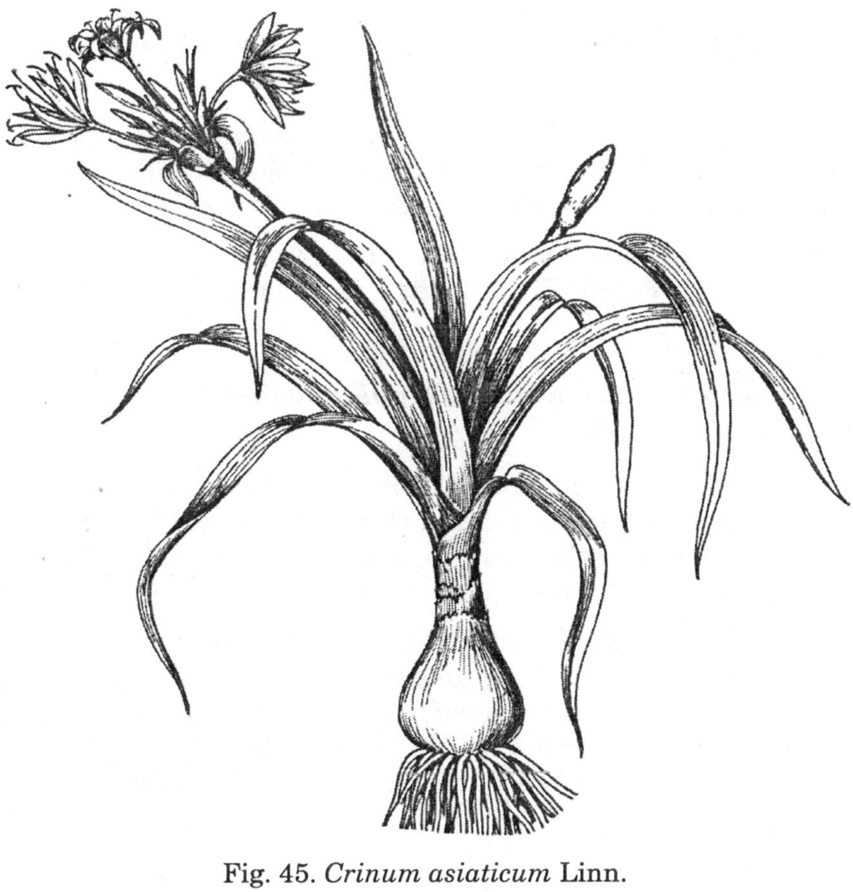

Fig. 45. *Crinum asiaticum* Linn.

Crotalaria burhia **Buch.-Ham. ex Benth (Fabaceae)** *Kharsana, Jhunda*

Low undershrub; branches numerous, stiff erectopatent, clothed with fine pale momentum; leaves simple, scattered, subsessile, rigid, pale green, 6- to 12-flowered, pedicels short; flowers yellow, small; pods oblong, 3- to 4-seeded. Characteristic wild desert plant of sand dunes. Fl. & Fr.: March – August.

Decoction of whole plant is given to animal to treat urinary problems and also for disposal of placenta after delivery. Extract of whole plant is given to treat constipation.

Crotalaria juncea **Linn. (Fabaceae)** *Sann, Sanai*

Shrub; leaves elliptic-lanceolate flowers yellow; fruits turgid, oblong. Cultivated during rainy season as a green manure crop and for fibres obtained from the stem Fl. & Fr.: September – February.

200 g boiled seeds are fed to animal to treat debility.

Cucumis callosus **(Rottl.) Cogn. (Cucurbitaceae)** *Kachra, Kachrio*

Perennial, trailing herb; leaves ovate-oblong or obovate; tendrils simple; flowers yellow; fruits obovoid, longitudinally variegated. Common in desertic zones. Fl. & Fr.: August – December.

Fruits are crushed and given to the animal with sugar, oil and water to treat diarrhoea. Fresh fruits are fed with fodder for disposal of placenta after delivery.

Curculigo orchioides **Gaertn. (Hypoxidaceae)** *Kali musli, Gocirari- dawai, Khajuri* (Plate 6)

Herbaceous plant, rootstock tuberous or elongated; leaves lanceolate, plicate, glabrous; scape 2.5 cm, clavate, flattened, hidden by leaf-sheath; flowers subsessile, lowest bisexual, rest male. Subtropical plant; wild. Fl. & Fr.: May-August.

Paste of 10 g tuberous roots of *Curculigo orchioides* is given orally along with water as an antidote to treat snake bite, scorpion bite, etc. Dried tubers of *Curculigo orchioides* are ground with stem of *Cissus quadrangularis* and given orally to treat impaction. Paste of root is fed to the animal with wheat bread to treat foot and mouth disease.

Curcuma amada **Roxb. (Zingiberaceae)** *Jangli haldi, Ambahaldi* (Plate 6)

Herb; rootstock ovoid, sessile tubers thick, pale yellow inside; leafy tuft, 60- 90 cm high, petiole as long as lamina, leaf blade pale green, tapering at the base and apex, scape from the center of the leafy tuft; spikes 7.5-15.0 cm by 3.7 cm, bracts pale green. Rare in the forest, so far reported only from the south-eastern parts of the state. Fl. & Fr.: August-September.

50 g dried rhizomes of *Curcuma amada,* 2 to 3 bulbs of *Allium cepa* and 500 g jaggery are mixed well and fed to the animal to treat indigestion and flatulence. Paste of 250 g of fresh rhizomes is given only once to treat fever.

About 100 g of dried rhizome powder of *Curcuma amada* is mixed with 100 g of rock salt, 100 g of alum, 100 g of *Piper longum,* 100 g of seeds of *Trachyspermum ammi,* 250 g jaggery and 100 g milk fat. This mixture is divided in 3 parts. One part is given once in a day for 3 days to treat gynecological problem after delivery, especially disposal of placenta after delivery.

Curcuma longa **Linn. (Zingiberaceae)** *Haldi, Haldu, Halad*

Rhizomes large, yielding turmeric; leaves oblong-elliptic; flowers pale-yellow. Cultivated for its edible rhizomes. Fl. & Fr.: October-February.

Paste of rhizome powder is applied with salt to treat sprains, swelling and mastitis.

Curcuma aromatica **Salisb. (Zingiberaceae)** *Haldi*

Erect, perennial herb, leaves elliptic or lanceolate – oblong. In moist and shady places in the forests. Fl. & Fr.: July – November.

Decoction prepared from the mixture of Alum (10g), powder of rhizomes of *Curcuma longa* (50g) and jaggery (2 kg) is given to animal for treatment of fractured bone. Extract of tuber is given to domestic animals orally through drenching tube in food poisoning. A mixture of seed oil of *Brassica campestris, 5* g rhizome of *Curcuma longa* and 2 g potash alum is given to the animal orally through a drenching tube to treat internal wound

Cuscuta reflexa **Roxb. (Cuscutaceae)** *Amar bel, Akash bel* (Plate 6)

A yellow, leafless, fleshy, twining parasite, branches stout, fleshy, forming dense yellow mass on shrubs and low trees; racemes lax, 2.5-

10.0 cm long, clustered or subspicate. Common throughout the state, usually parasitising on *Adhatoda zeylanica, Acacia nilotica, Ziziphus nummularia* and *Ziziphus mauritiana.* Fl. & Fr.: October- January.

1 kg whole plant of *Cuscuta reflexa,* 1kg leaves of *Datura innoxia* are boiled in one litre of mustard oil. Massage of this oil is given to the animal to treat lumbago and rheumatic pain. About 400 - 500 g of fresh stem is mixed with animal feed to treat haematuria.

***Cyamopsis tetragonoloba* (Linn.) Taub. (Fabaceae)** *Gawar*

Erect, robust annual, 30-60 cm high, clothed with appressed greying hairs, stem grooved, leaves trifoliate, flowers small, purplish in axillary racemes, fruits thick fleshy pods, in clusters, subtetragonal, more or less hairy; seeds 5-12 in each pod, compressed to some extent. Commonly cultivated during rainy season for its edible pods and as a fodder crop. Fl. & Fr.: July- November.

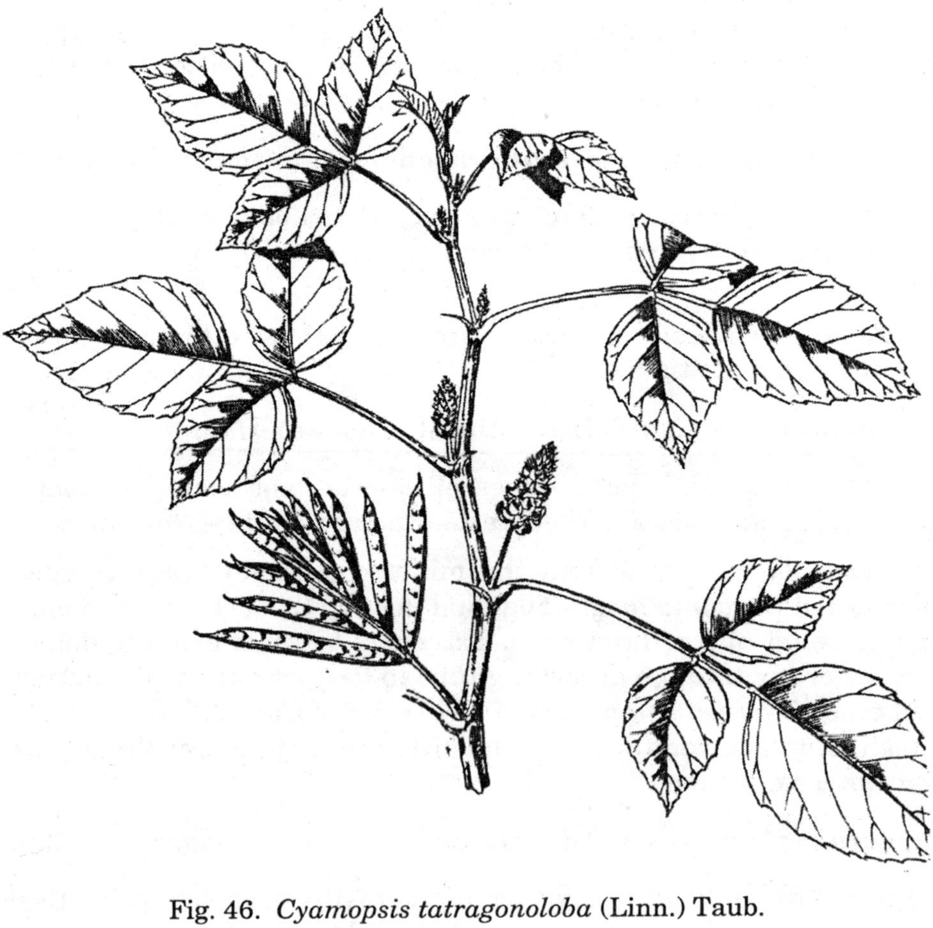

Fig. 46. *Cyamopsis tatragonoloba* (Linn.) Taub.

Fruits and seeds of this plant are given with fodder to the animal to treat diarrhoea. 100 gm of this mixture is also given to the animal with pearl millet grains for disposal of the placenta after the delivery.

Cymbopogon martinii **(Roxb.) Wats. (Poaceae)** *Rhodo, Chant* (Plate 6)

Perennial, sweet-scented grass, 1.5-2.5 m high; leaves linear-lanceolate, sub- cordate, amplexicaul and finely cordate; flowers in panicled spikelets, turning reddish brown when mature, glumes channelled corresponding to a midrib on the inner side, awned. Prefers drier soils. Fl. & Fr.: August-December.

Fumigation of whole plant is given to the animal to treat fever.

Dalbergia sissoo **Roxb. (Fabaceae)** *Sisham, Talli*

Deciduous tree, with 3-5 acuminate leaflets; flowers yellowish in axillary panicles; pods oblong or strap shaped, flat narrowed at the base. Common in wastelands, along the roads, boundaries of fields and gardens. Fl. & Fr.: March-August.

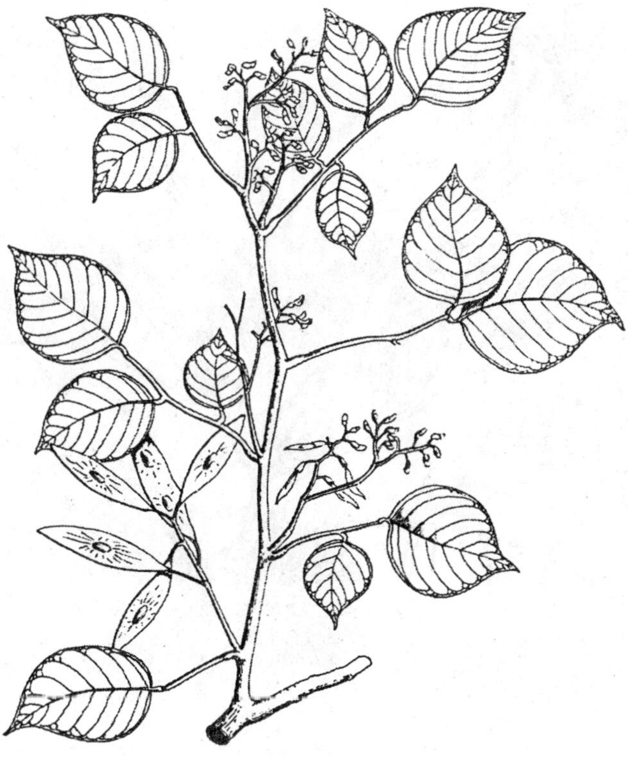

Fig. 47. *Dalbergia sissoo* Roxb.

Paste of about 250 g leaves of *Dalbergia sissoo* is given to the animal with drenching tube to treat diarrhoea. Oil is extracted through traditional method by heating bark of *Dalbergia sissoo* mixed with hard coconut shell and applied in small quantity to treat eczema, abscess or septic wound. Large amount causes burning sensation. Infusion of 2 kg leaves is given to camel to treat sunstroke. Leaves of *Dalbergia sissoo* are soaked overnight in water and given in the morning orally to the camel to treat dysuria.

***Datura innoxia* Mill. (Solanaceae)** *Dhatura*

Stout shrub, upto 1 m high, clothed with grey pubescence; leaves ovate, sinuate-toothed; flowers axillary, solitary; pedicels 2-3 cm long, recurved in fruit; capsules 3.5-5.5 cm in diameter, globose, densely pubescent and armed with weak, 1.0-1.8 cm long spines. Common in wasteland, especially in the east of Aravalli. Fl. & Fr.: Most part of the year.

The paste of whole plant is applied locally to treat mastitis whereas powder of seeds is given to animal to treat oestrus induction.

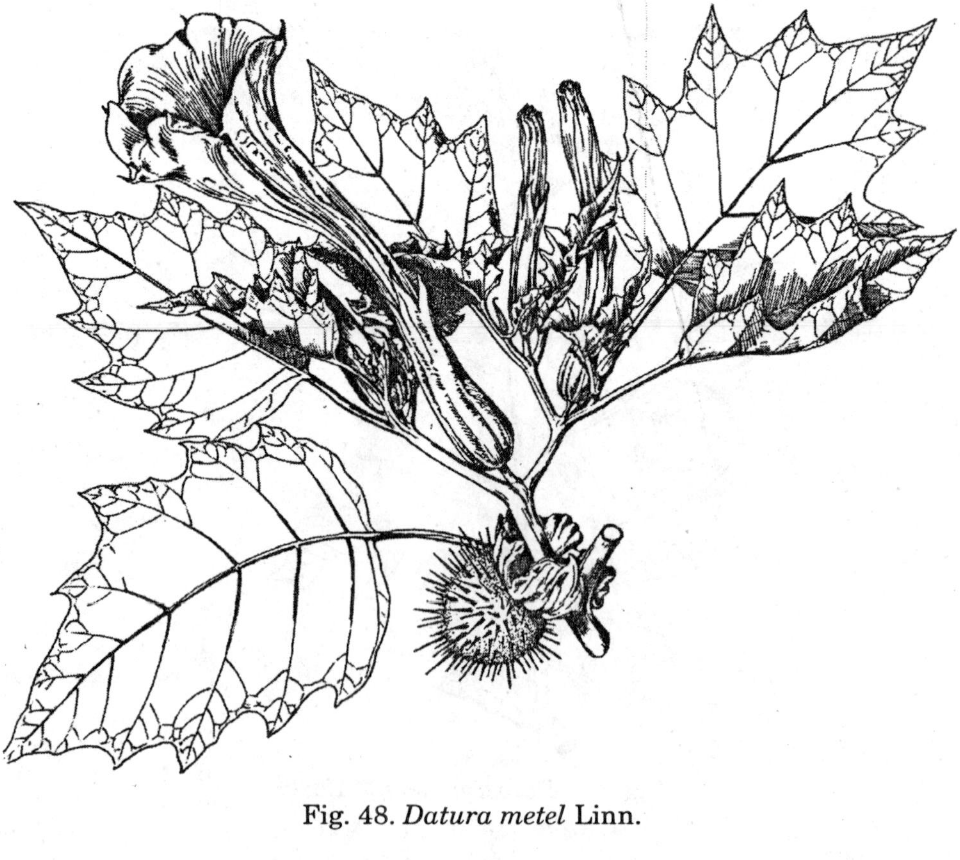

Fig. 48. *Datura metel* Linn.

Datura metel **Linn. (Solanaceae)** *Dhatura, Kala- dhatura*

Herb; leaves triangular, ovate; flowers axillary, solitary; capsule subglobose, deflexed, clothed with blunt tubercles. Naturalized in wastelands and open forests. Fl. & Fr.: Most part of the year.

Extract of fresh leaves is given to the animal twice a day for 3 days to treat tonsillitis.

Delonix elata **(Linn.) Gamble (Caesalpiniaceae)** *Sandeshra*

Tall, erect, deciduous tree; leaves 4-15 cm long; pinnae 4-6 pairs; flowers in terminal racemes; pods linear-oblanceolate, reticulate, beaked, glabrous, dark brown. Common in wastelands; also planted along the roadsides. Fl. & Fr.: November - June.

Decoction of 100 gm crushed stem bark is given to animal to treat dysentery and diarrhoea.

Dendrocalamus strictus **(Roxb.) Nees (Poaceae)** *Bans, Vanhedo*

Densely tufted, arborescent bamboos, upto 10 m tall, with swollen nodes; lower stem- sheaths covered on the back with golden- brown stiff hairs; internodes upto 50 cm long; ligules narrow, serrate; inflorescence a panicle of dense, globular heads; caryopsis subglobose, brown. Fairly common in dry deciduous forests on the top of hills forming distant patches. Fl. & Fr.: At the interval of many years.

Infusion of tender stem is given to animal once in a day upto three days to treat fractured bone. One tender culm (about 25-30 cm in length) is crushed and given to the animal orally two to three times to remove the intestinal worms. Decoction of stem is given to the animal for disposal of placenta after delivery.

Dendrophthoe falcata **(L. f.) Etting (Loranthaceae)** *Kavlate ke bel, Salar-bel, Banda* (Plate 6)

Dichotomously branched, partial stem- parasite; with elliptic-oblong, obovate or ovate- lanceolate leaves; flowers red, orange or yellowish-red in unilateral spikes; berries ovoid. A common stem parasite on the branches of *Boswellia serrata* and *Commiphora wightii* in hilly tracts. Fl. & Fr.: August-February.

Extract of whole plant is applied locally on uterus to treat vulvo-vaginal-uterine -prolapse.

***Desmostachya bipinnata* (Linn.) Stapf (Poaceae)** *Dabb, Dabra*

Tufted, stout, erect, rhizomatous perennial, upto 1.25m tall; with creeping root- stocks; leaves acuminate, sheaths glabrous, densely flagellate; inflorescence 25- 50 cm long, spikes 1.5-3.5 cm long, cluster bearing 20-30 spikelets, spikelets 2.5- 3.5 mm long, linear, oblong, glumes unequal, lemmas 2.5mm long, straw coloured. Commonly found near moist places particularly in sandy and clayey soils. Fl. & Fr.: July-November.

Whole plant is fed to the animal to treat dysentery.

***Dichrostachys cinerea* (Linn.) Wt. & Arn. (Mimosaceae)** *Ameena, Goya- Khair*

Polygamous shrub; branchlets usually ending in spines, pubescent; leaves 2-pinnate, upto 6.5 cm long, with stalk, stipiform glands at the insertion of pinnae; spikes axillary or extra axillary; pods 4-7 by 0.6 0 -1.0 cm, compressed, pubescent, dark brown. Common in open forests on rocky and sandy- loam soil. Fl. & Fr.: July – November.

Seeds are boiled and given to the animal to treat hypogalactia.

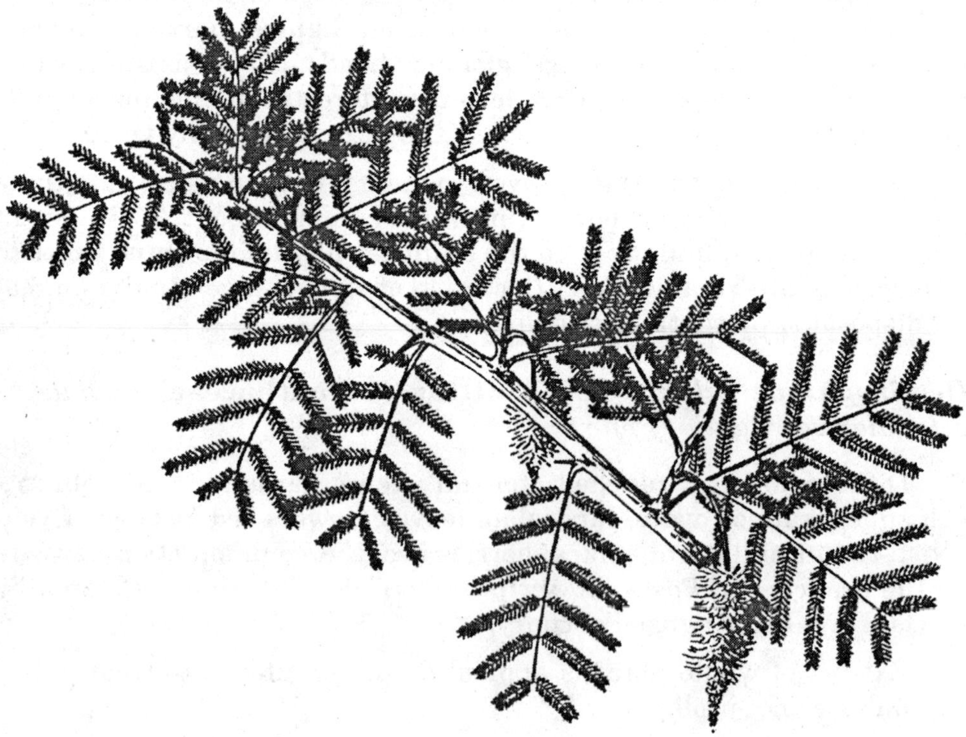

Fig. 49. *Dichrostachys cinerea* (Linn.) Wt. & Arn.

Digitaria adscendens **(H.B. & K.) Henr. (Poaceae)** *Ghass*

Erect or geniculately ascending annuals, often rooting at the lower nodes; leaves linear lanceolate; racemes 3-9, subsessile, subdigitate, 5-20 cm long; spikelets 2-nate. Fairly common throughout the state as forest undergrowth, in wastelands and neglected places. Fl. & Fr.: August – October.

Mixture of seeds of *Digitaria adscendens, Tribulus terrestris, Cucumis melo, Pedalium murex* and *Citrullus lanatus* is given to the animal to treat constipation.

Dioscorea alata **Linn. (Dioscoreaceae)** *Kada – kanda, Ratalu*

Climbing or twining herbs, with large tuberous roots; stem 4-angled; leaves cordate-ovate to cordate-oblong; male flowers green, in panicles; female flowers in simple spikes; capsules leathery, elliptic, 3-winged. Mostly cultivated for its edible tubers. Fl. & Fr.: August–December.

For treating all kind of abscesses in the animals, tubers of *Dioscorea alata* are fed to the animal.

Dioscorea bulbifera **Linn. (Dioscoreaceae)** *Vahrikand, Jangli aritha, Modi, Ratha sankriyo, Raalar* (Plate 6)

Twining, dioecious, glabrous herb with globose or pyriform tubers; bulbils common in leaf - axils; leaves alternate, broadly ovate- cordate to suborbicular, acute to acuminate, entire, 7 to 13 nerved at the base; male flowers closely arranged in long, pendulous simple or paniculate spikes; female flowers subtended by minute bracts in axillary, solitary or fascicled, pendulous spikes; seeds winged on the basal side only. Common in wastelands and open forests among bushes and shrubs and along hedges. Fl. & Fr.: August-December.

Paste of 25-30 g tuber is given to the animal once in a day to treat mastitis. Larger quantity is poisonous.Tuberous roots are fed to the animal to treat sterility.

Diospyros melanoxylon **Roxb. (Ebenaceae)** *Tendu, Timru, Tendu-patta*

Deciduous tree, bark exfoliating in 4- angular scales; leaves 5.17 by 4-12 cm, ovate- elliptic or oblong, coriaceous, pubescent; male flowers in subsessile, drooping cymes, female flowers solitary; fruits 2-4 cm in diameter; seeds obovate oblong, blackish. Fairly common in the forest and wastelands. Fl. & Fr.: April- November.

Crushed fruits are given to the animal to treat dysentery.

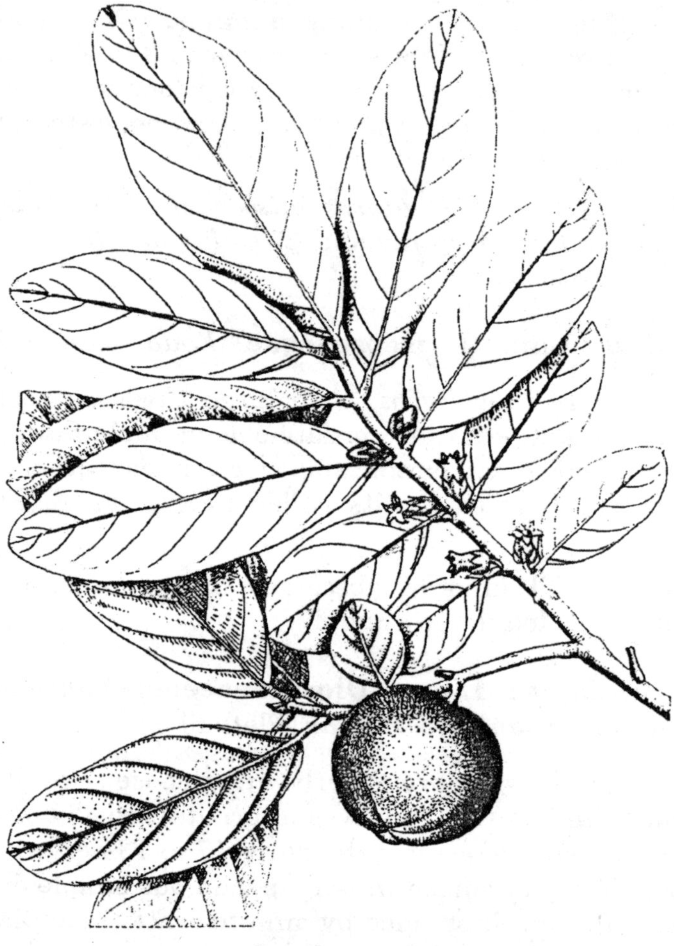

Fig. 50. *Diospyros melanoxylon* Roxb.

***Echinops echinatus* Roxb. (Asteraceae)** *Modokanto, Oont-Kantalo, Oont- kanti, Utkali*

White cottony herbs; with pinnatifid, spinescent leaves; heads white, blue or yellow, 1- flowered, clustered in spinous globose compound heads. Common on sandy plains and dunes, rarely on hard gravel soils. Fl. & Fr.: October- June.

Infusion of roots is given to animal to treat flatulence whereas extract of roots is applied locally on the uterus to treat vulvo-vaginal-uterine- prolapse. About 100 g of root powder of *Echinops echinatus* and 100 g bark powder of *Acacia senegal* are mixed in 1 kg curd and applied twice in a day on the body of animal to remove lice and ticks.

Elettaria cardamomum **Maton (Zingiberaceae)** *Elaichi*

A tall herbaceous perennial with subterranean branching rootstock, 1.5 to 5 m in height; leaves subsessile, elliptic or lanceolate with sheathing base; flower in panicles; fruits trilocular, subglobose capsule, marked with many vertical ribs; seeds 15-20 per pod. Cultivated plant. Fl. & Fr.: September – January.

Dry seed powder is mixed with clove and fed to the animal for disposal of placenta after delivery.

Eleusine coracana **(Linn.) Gaertn. (Poaceae)** *Maal*

Tall, erect, stout annuals; leaves distichous, flat, linear, acute; ligule a hairy membrane; spikes digitate; rachis flattened; caryopsis smooth and rugose Mostly cultivated in the eastern Rajasthan for its edible grains.Fl. & Fr.: August – November.

Bread made up of *Eleusine coracana* flour is fed to the animal once in a day to treat diarrhoea and twice a day to treat mastitis locally called as "*thanella*".

Elytraria acaulis **(L.f.) Lind. (Acanthaceae)** *Kala gathia, Galobi, Dasmul*

Herb, upto 20 cm high, with fibrous roots; leaves obovate to oblanceolate, rounded or obtuse, crenate, base cuneate, glabrous, scapes upto 22 cm long, many flowers in simple or branched spikes; fruit white; capsule 0.5- 0.75 by 0.25- 0.35 cm, ovoid, acute, glabrous, brownish; seeds many, more or less ovoid, minute, flattened, papillose brown. Common in moist and shady places viz. rock- crevices, along the streams and other rocky gravelly habitats. Fl. & Fr.: April-October.

Decoction of 50 g of dried roots is given to the animal twice in a day for 7 days to treat nematoid infection. Extract of whole plant is given to animal to treat dysentery.

Enicostema axillare **(Lam.) Raynal (Gentianaceae)** *Naame, Naama, Kadava, Nahli* (Plate 6)

Perennial herb, with quadrangular branches from the base; leaves sessile, 1-7 by 0.6-1.3 cm, linear to linear lanceolate, obtuse, amplexicaule; flowers subsessile, many in axillary, capitate, opposite fascicles, white; capsule 3- 5 mm long, ellipsoid-oblong, glabrous, septicidally 2-valved; seeds many, minute. Common in open plains, forests, grassland and in cultivated field. Fl. & Fr.: September- January.

About 50 g leaves are given with fodder to the young animal upto five days to treat fever. Root extract is given orally and also applied locally on uterus of animal to treat vulvo - vaginal - uterine-prolapse.

***Ephedra ciliata* Fisch. & Mey. Ex C.A. Mey. (Gnetaceae)** *Oont phog*

Dioecious, much – branched, climbing or scandent shrubs; leaves 2-4 at each node, upto 25 by 1.5 mm long; fruits 8 by 7 mm, white, semi- transparent; seeds 2, brown. Generally found in desert on sandy to gravelly or even on rocky plains. Fl. & Fr.: January- April.

Decoction of about 5 kg plant is given to the animal to treat constipation.

***Euphorbia caducifolia* Haines (Euphorbiaceae)** *Thor*

Glabrous, perennial, fleshy shrub; stem armed with spines; leaves deciduous; cyathia in triads, red; styles bifid. Abundant in rocky habitats of Aravalli. Fl. & Fr.: January – April.

The latex of the plant is applied on uterus of animal to treat vulvo-vaginal - uterine - prolapse.

***Euphorbia fusiformis* Buch. - Ham. (Euphorbiaceae)** *Jangli palak, Pahadi mooli* (Plate 6)

Dwarf, glabrous herb; stem reduced to a long, stout, underground cylindric rootstock; leaves subsessile, ovate or oblanceolate; cyme from the crown of the rootstock, dichotomously branched, 3- to many flowered, appearing after the leaves have fallen; capsules 8 mm. in diameter, cocci compressed. Rare, in wastelands, particularly in the Southern parts of Rajasthan. Fl. & Fr.: April – June.

150 g tuber is crushed and given orally to the animal to treat sunstroke. Root powder is given orally to treat dysentery and fever.

***Euphorbia heyneana* Spreng. (Euphorbiaceae)** *Choti dudhee*

Prostrate, dichotomously branched, glabrous herb, with ribbed internodes; leaves opposite, obliquely oblong or obovate - oblong; cyathia reddish green; involucre stalked, axillary, campanulate, glabrous; capsule obtusely keeled glabrous. Common on rock crevices and marshy places Fl. & Fr.: October – March.

Whole plant is crushed and given to the animal along with fodder to stop excessive bleeding after delivery.

Euphorbia hirta **Linn. (Euphorbiaceae)** *Dudhi*

Procumbent, ascending or erect, annual, hairy herbs; leaves opposite, variable in size, obliquely lanceolate, ovate or rhomboid – oblong, stipules subulate; cyathia many, crowded in axillary and terminal, shortly pedunculate cymes; capsules globosely trigonous, appressedly hairy; seeds ovoid. Common throughout the state of Rajasthan, preferably in sandy habitats. Fl. & Fr.: Almost throughout the year.

Paste of about 25 g whole plant of *Euphorbia hirta* is given to the animal with water through drenching tube once only to treat diarrhoea. Paste of leaves of this plant and *Cynodon dactylon* is also given to the animal with milk to treat diarhoea.

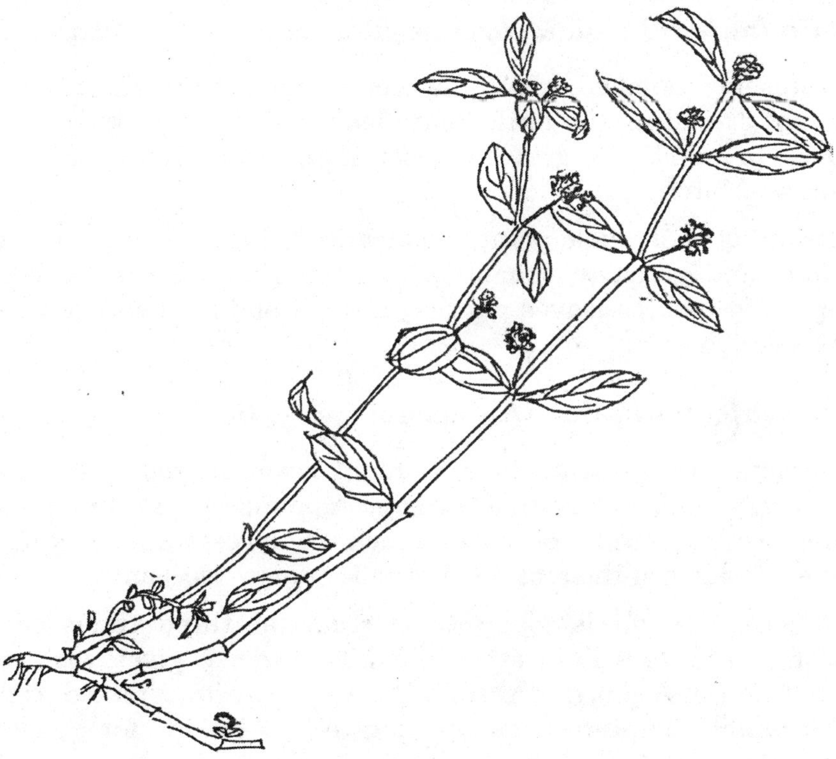

Fig. 51. *Euphorbia hirta* Linn.

Euphorbia neriifolia **Linn. (Euphorbiaceae)** *Danda - thor, Thuar*

Erect, deciduous shrub or small trees; leaves obovate-oblong, crowded at the stem; stem subfleshy; involucre 3 - nate; glands without petaloid limb. Common in rocky habitats in plains or on naked hillocks. Fl. & Fr.: March – July.

Two to three drops of the fresh latex of the plant is dropped over the injured portion as an antiseptic. Roots are fed to the cattle with fodder for oestrus induction and also disposal of placenta after delivery. Small quantity (4-5 drops) of latex is used as purgative to treat constipation.

***Euphorbia tirucalli* Linn. (Euphorbiaceae)** *Anguli thor*

Shrub or small tree; branches smooth, spreading, terete, rush like, almost leafless. Cultivated as hedge plant. Fl. & Fr.: September – December.

Latex is applied locally to treat skin diseases like dermatitis, eczema, etc.

***Fagonia indica* Burm. f. (Zygophyllaceae)** *Dhamasa*

Profusely branched, glandular herbs, with terete internodes and spines not exceeding the unifoliolate leaves; flowers pinkish – purple. Common in sandy to gravelly soils in desertic zones. Fl. & Fr.: September-March.

About 200 g of whole plant is boiled in 10 litre water till it reduces to 1 litre and given to camel to treat cough. Plant is boiled after adding 200 g tobacco leaves powder, filtered and applied externally to kill the lices.

***Ferula asafoetida* Linn. (Apiaceae)** *Hing*

Perennial herbs, upto to 2 m high; lower leaves ovate, cauline sheath large; umbels terminal, large, compound. vittae broad, as long as the carples; seeds dorsally much compressed. Cultivated for resinous exudates of the root. Fl. & Fr.: January – December.

10 g Asafoetida is given to the animal three times to treat infection of nematode in intestines. Resin powder is given with milk to treat flatulence. A pinch of resin of *Ferula asafoetida* mixed with 500 ml of *Brassica campestris* seed oil is given to buffalo for quick relief from flatulence.

***Ficus benghalensis* Linn. (Moraceae)** *Badd, Bargad, Vad, Vadlo, Badla*

Large evergreen tree, with prop roots and grey to greyish brown, rough bark; leaves alternate, ovate-oblong, ovate - orbicular or elliptic, coriaceous; receptacles axillary, geminate, depressed - globose, silky - pubescent, bright red when ripe. Common in wastelands, walls of old buildings and on other trees, also planted as an avenue tree along roads and near the temples. Fl. & Fr.: Almost throughout the year.

Paste of bark and root is applied to treat the fractured bone.

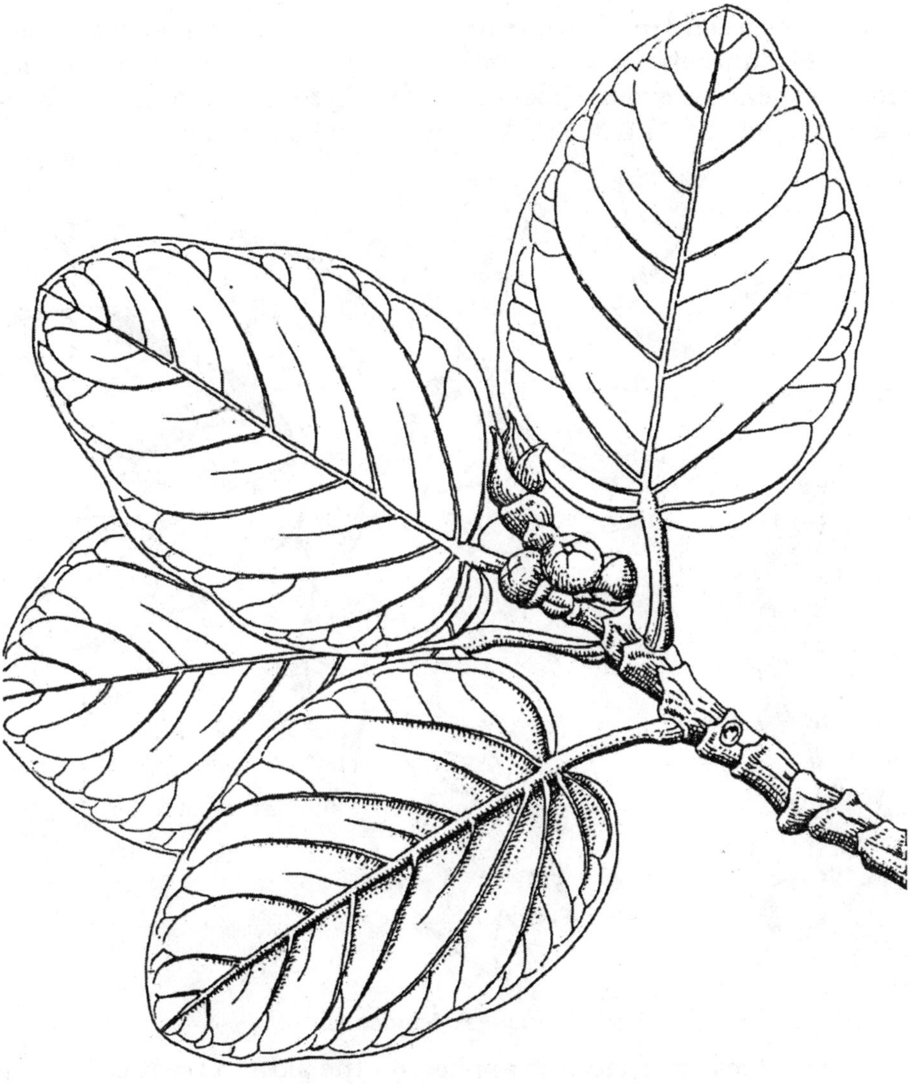

Fig. 52. *Ficus benghalensis* Linn.

***Ficus carica* Linn. (Moraceae)** *Anjir*

Tall tree, without aerial roots; leaves broadly ovate, entire or lobed, softly pubescent beneath; receptacles axillary, obovoid oblong, thinly pubescent. Cultivated for its sweet, edible figs used as dry fruits. Fl. & Fr.: Throughout the year.

Latex of *Ficus carica* is applied on the skin to treat eczema and carbuncles.

***Ficus racemosa* Linn. (Moraceae)** *Gular, Umar, Umbio, Kusumati*

Tall evergreen tree, with short aerial roots; leaves ovate - oblong or elliptic- lanceolate; receptacles on short, warted, tuberculate, leafless branchlets, ovoid; achenes reddish-brown. Found in the forests along water courses. Fl. & Fr.: Almost throughout the year.

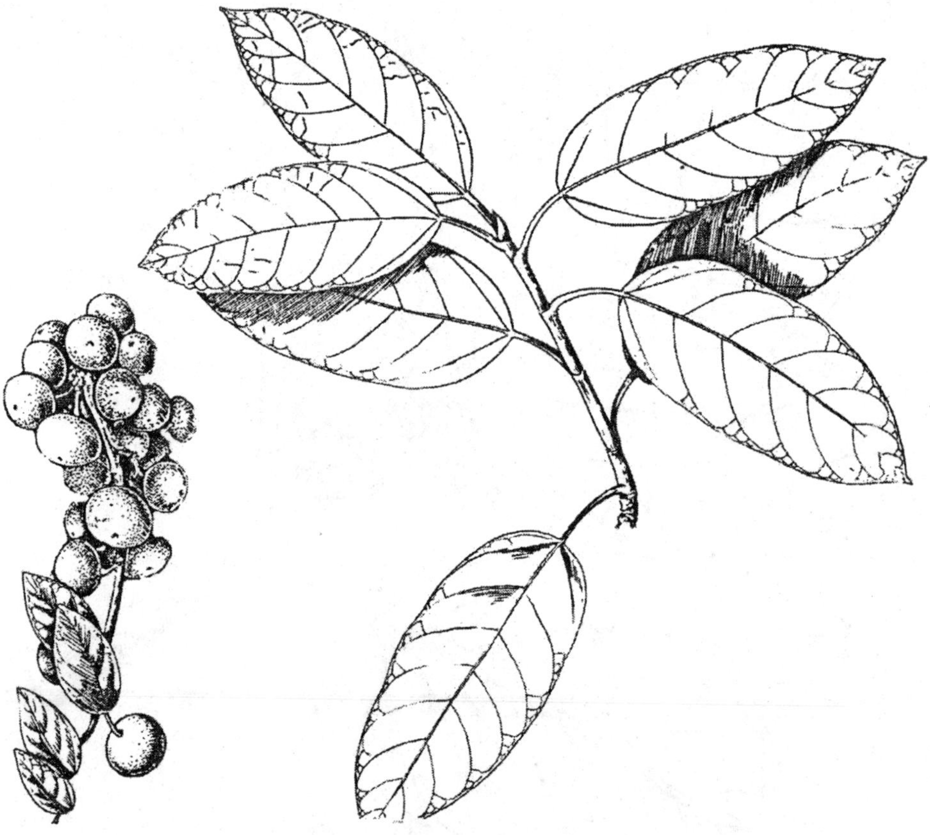

Fig. 53. *Ficus racemosa* Linn.

Latex of *Ficus racemosa* is applied on the skin to treat carbuncles. Paste of bark of *Ficus racemosa* is applied on the injury caused by snake-bite. Few drops of latex of the plant is applied locally on skin as an antiseptic.

***Ficus religiosa* Linn. (Moraceae)** *Pipal, Peepli*

Large, deciduous, glabrous tree, with grey or grayish black bark; leaves ovate - suborbicular; receptacles in axillary pairs, spherical, reddish purple when ripe. Common in wastelands, on the walls of old buildings, on large trees and usually planted near temples all over the area. Fl. & Fr.: Almost throughout the year.

Extract of about 5 kg leaves of this plant is given orally to the buffalo after giving bath to treat dysuria and haematuria. Decoction of bark is given to the animal for disposal of placenta after delivery. 250 g crushed fruits are given to the animal to conceive.

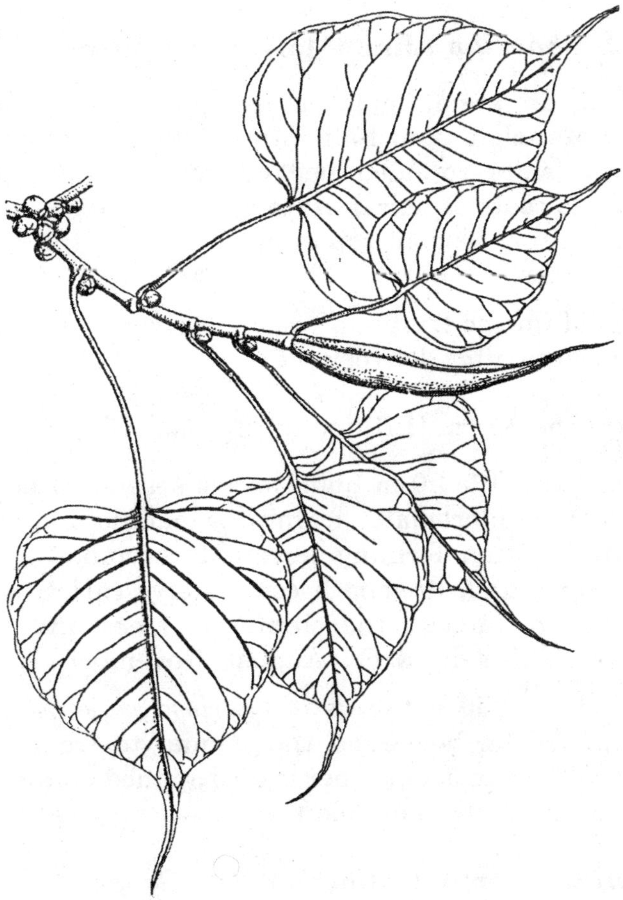

Fig. 54. *Ficus religiosa* Linn.

***Gardenia turgida* Roxb. (Rutaceae)** *Padairi, Padatatu*

Small, deciduous tree; branches armed with straight thorns; leaves elliptic to obovate, entire, glabrous; flowers from the young leafless shoots, white, unisexual, male fascicled, female solitary. Occasional in the forests. Fl. & Fr.: April – June.

Leaf decoction is applied locally to treat the wound.

Garuga pinnata Roxb. (Burseraceae) *Kankad, Vanagra*

Tall deciduous tree, 7-15 m high; leaves crowded at the end of branches, 20 - 36 cm long; leaflets 11-21, sessile, elliptic oblong, pubescent beneath; flowers in 7-20 cm long, terminal panicles, creamy white; drupes subpyriform, fleshy, smooth, glabrous. Rare, in dry deciduous forest. Fl. & Fr.: January - May.

Decoction of bark is used to treat the infection in hooves.

Gossypium herbaceum Linn. (Malvaceae) *Kapas*

A small shrub; stem rigid sparsely pilose and branched; leaves simple, alternate, cleft upto half into 3-7 lobes; flowers yellow with purple centre; fruits rounded beaked capsules, 3-4 locular, seeds usually with two coats of hairs, white grey or reddish brown in colour. Cultivated as a rainy season crop in many parts of the state. Fl. & Fr.: August – November.

Decoction of unripe fruits and roots is given to the animal for the disposal of placenta after delivery.

Gloriosa superba Linn. (Liliaceae) *Kalihari* (Plate 7)

Perennial herb, 1.5-4.0 m high; leaves sessile, alternate, opposite or in whorls, ovate - lanceolate, acuminate, ending in a tendril; flowers axillary, solitary, often forming terminal corymbose, yellow, tinged with red in upper half, at length completely scarlet; capsule oblong septicidal. Common among the clumps of trees and shrubs in the forests of Aravalli hills. Fl. & Fr.: August- November.

Paste of about 250 g tubers of *Gloriosa superba* is mixed with water and applied on hooves of the animal to treat from foot and mouth disease. The extract of tuber is also applied on uterus of animals to treat vulvo-vaginal uterine-prolapse.

Grewia damine Gaertn. (Tiliaceae) *Gangestri*

Shrub, young parts tomentose; leaves ovate - oblong; flowers in axillary, umbellate cymes. Rare, in wastelands and open forests. Fl. & Fr.: January – October.

About 50 g roots are crushed and given with water, twice in a day upto three days to treat fractured bone. The extract of leaves, 4 to 5 eggs of hen and milk of cow is mixed and given to the animal daily with the help of either a tumbler or drenching tube upto 10 days to treat fractured bone.

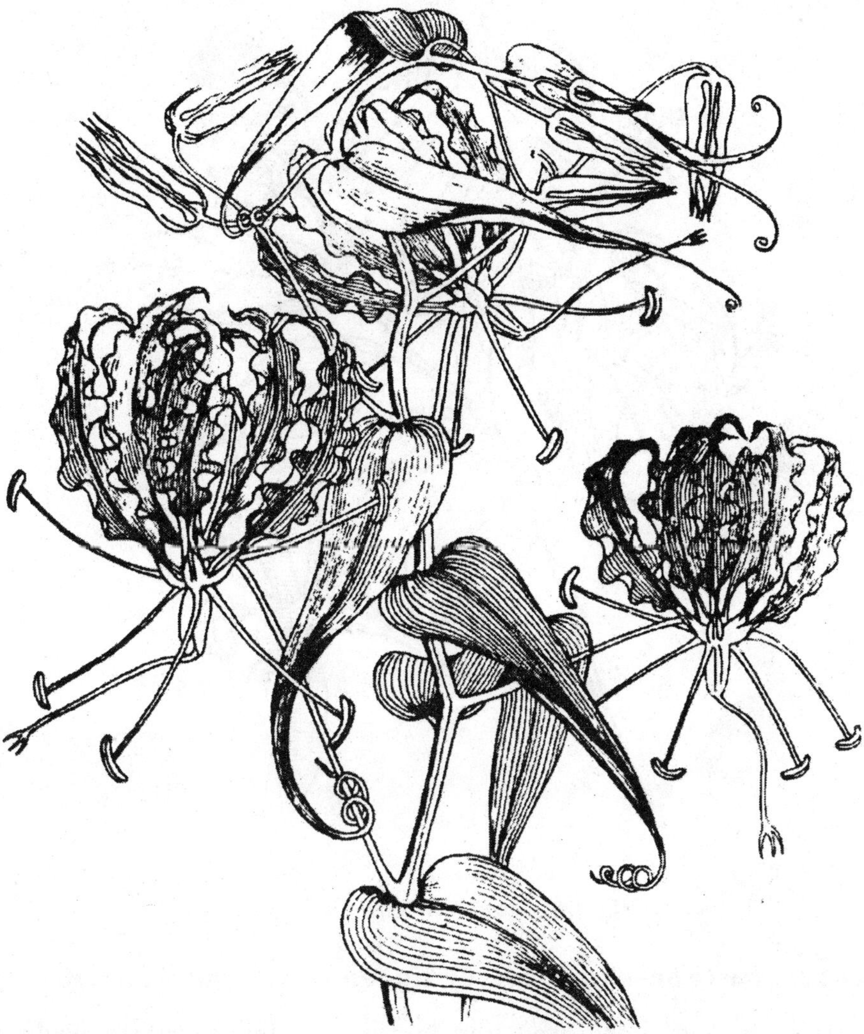

Fig. 55. *Gloriosa superba* Linn.

***Grewia orientalis* Linn. (Tiliaceae)** *Gangchi*

Large shrub or small tree; leaves elliptic - oblong to sub - orbicular; flowers in axillary cymes; drupes 8 -10 mm in diameter, subglobose, 2 to 4 - lobed, hairy when young. Rare, in scrub forests. Fl. & Fr.: September – October.

About 50 g leaves are fed to the animal with fodder to treat impaction. 50 g root powder is mixed with 500 ml water and given with cold water to treat stomach disorder. Root extract of *Grewia orientalis* is given orally to treat fractured bone.

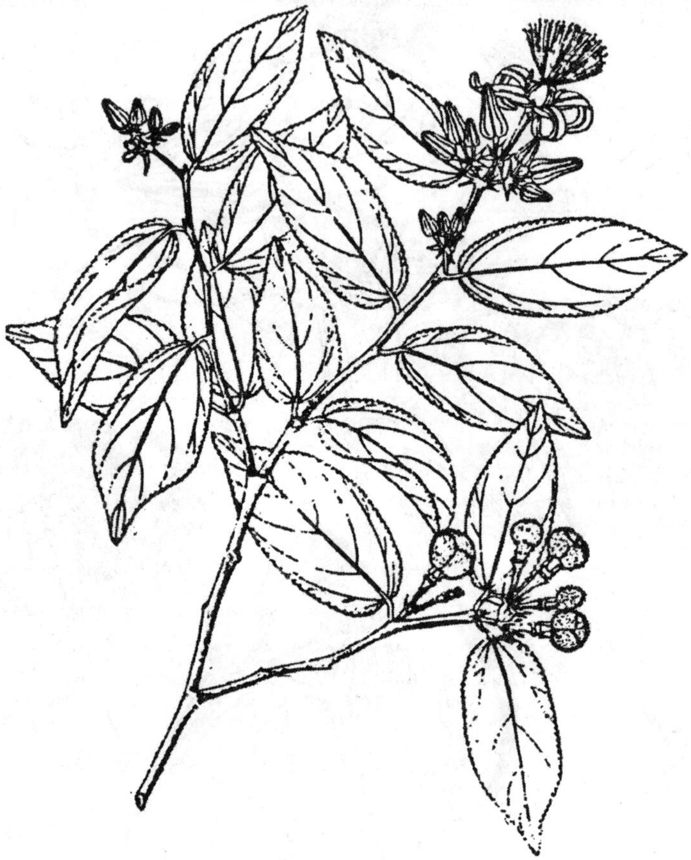

Fig. 56. *Grewia orientalis* Linn.

Grewia tenax **(Forssk.) Fiori. (Tiliaceae)** *Gangir, Kankera*

Shrub, bark ash-coloured and lenticelled; leaves ovate-cordate or ovate-oblong, crenate, glabrous above, hairy beneath; flowers in pedunculate, umbellate cyme; drupes 1.0-1.5 cm in diam., 2 to 4 - lobed, glabrous, orange coloured when ripe; stones 1-4, 1 to 2 celled. Common in the forests, on the hill slopes, wastelands and on the boundaries of fields and gardens. Fl. & Fr.: August – October.

Root powder is given to the animal to treat fractured bone.

Guizotia oleifera **DC. (Asteraceae)** *Kali teeli*

A stout, erect, smooth or scabrid, leafy herb; leaves sessile, half - amplexicaul, linear or lanceolate - oblong, obtuse, serrate; head 1.2 - 2.5 cm in diam.; peduncle naked. Grows as a weed in cultivated fields. Fl. & Fr.: September – December.

Poultice of leaves is tied locally (on the swollen portion of animal body) to get rid of swelling with pain.

Helicteres isora **Linn. (Sterculiaceae)** *Marorphalli, Hateri* (Plate 7)

Shrub or small tree; leaves bifarious, broadly ovate to orbicular; flowers solitary or in few - flowered axillary cymes. Common in forests, particularly on hilly slopes. Fl. & Fr.: August – November.

Powder of 100 g pods is given orally to animal to treat dysentery. About 100 g paste either of bark or dried seeds of *Helicterus isora* are given thrice in a day upto three days to treat in bloody dysentery and diarrhoea.

Hemidesmus indicus **(Linn.) R. Br. (Periplocaceae)** *Dudhli, Garmali, Anantmul, Koorvi*

Scandent undershrub, with woody rootstock, leaves opposite, elliptic - oblong to linear - lanceolate, acute at the apex; flowers in axillary, subsessile cyme; follicles tapering to a joint, slightly falcate, glabrous; seeds, ovate oblong, compressed, black. Common in forest in south-east of Aravalli. Fl. & Fr.: Almost throughout the year.

Root decoction is applied locally to treat skin diseases.

Heteropogon contortus **(Linn.) P. Beauv. (Poaceae)** *Suva ghass, Lapida, Lapia, Pallio, Lapadioo*

Erect, tufted perennial; leaves, linear, acuminate, sheaths compressed, keeled, glabrous; ligule a ciliate, scarious rim; racemes solitary; spikelets closely imbricate; lower glumes of sessile spikelets long, elliptic - oblong, hispidulous awn long, hirtellous. Fairly common in south-eastern Rajasthan in open wastelands, fallow fields, along roadsides etc. Fl. & Fr.: August – November.

The whole plant is crushed and given orally to animal to treat constipation.

Hibiscus rosa- sinensis **Linn. (Malvaceae)** *Gurhal*

Evergreen shrubs; flowers axillary, pink, red or rose-coloured; staminal tube exceeding the corolla. Fl. & Fr.: Throughout year.

About 500 g leaves of *Hibiscus rosa- sinensis* are fed to the animal with fodder to treat haematuria and leucorrhoea.

Holarrhena pubescens **(Buch.-Ham.) Wall. ex G. Don (Apocynaceae)** *Kadi, Kodaya, Hadadiyo, Kadwa*

Shrub or small tree; leaves ovate - elliptic abruptly acuminate; flowers white in corymbose cymes, follicles cylindric, lenticelled; seed linear - oblong compressed, comose. Common in the forest in hilly tracts. Fl. & Fr.: May – September.

Extract of stem bark is given orally to the animal to treat dysentery and anthrax. Stem bark paste is applied locally to treat wound.

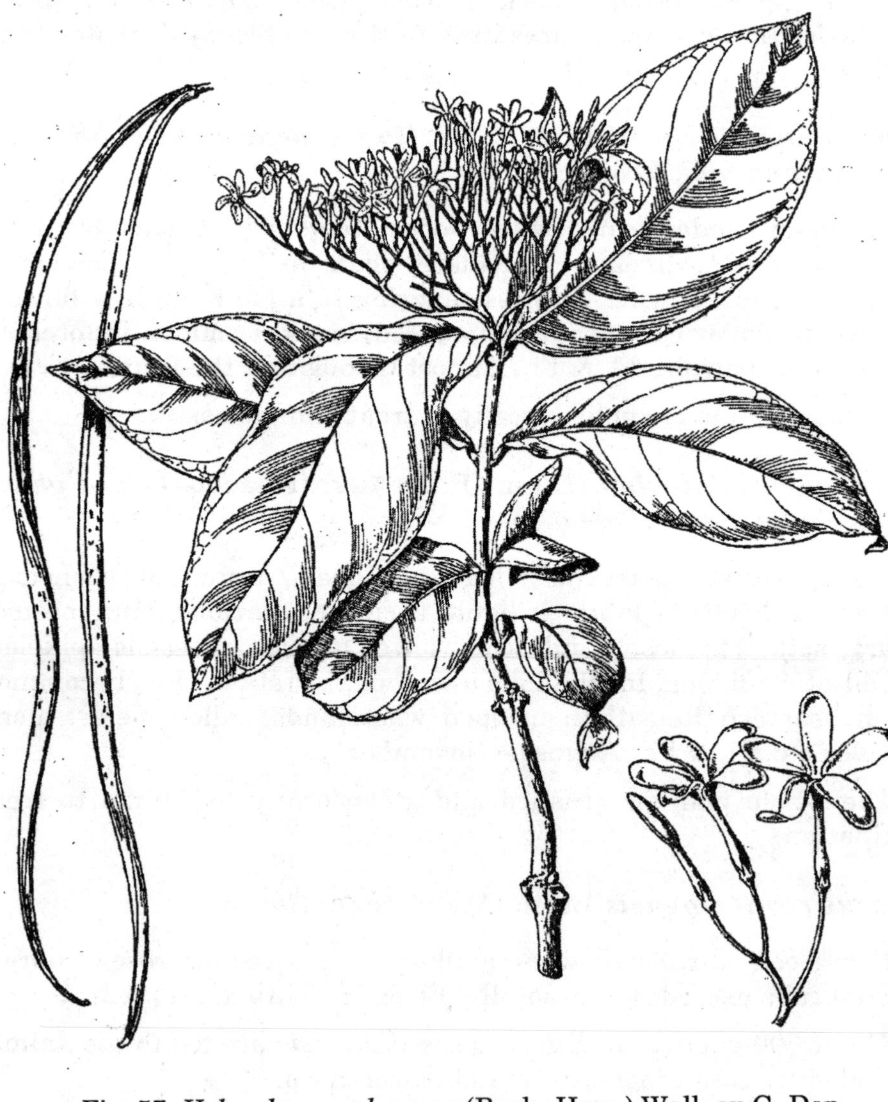

Fig. 57. *Holarrhena pubescens* (Buch.-Ham.) Wall. ex G. Don

Holoptelea integrifolia **(Roxb.) Planch. (Ulmaceae)** *Bander bati, Churil*

Large, spreading, almost glabrous, deciduous tree; leaves ovate to abruptly acuminate; flowers greenish - yellow; fruits broadly oblong or orbicular, deeply notched at the apex, flat, winged. Common in the dry deciduous forests, wastelands etc. Fl. & Fr.: December – May.

Paste of leaves of *Holoptelea integrifolia* is applied to treat eczema.

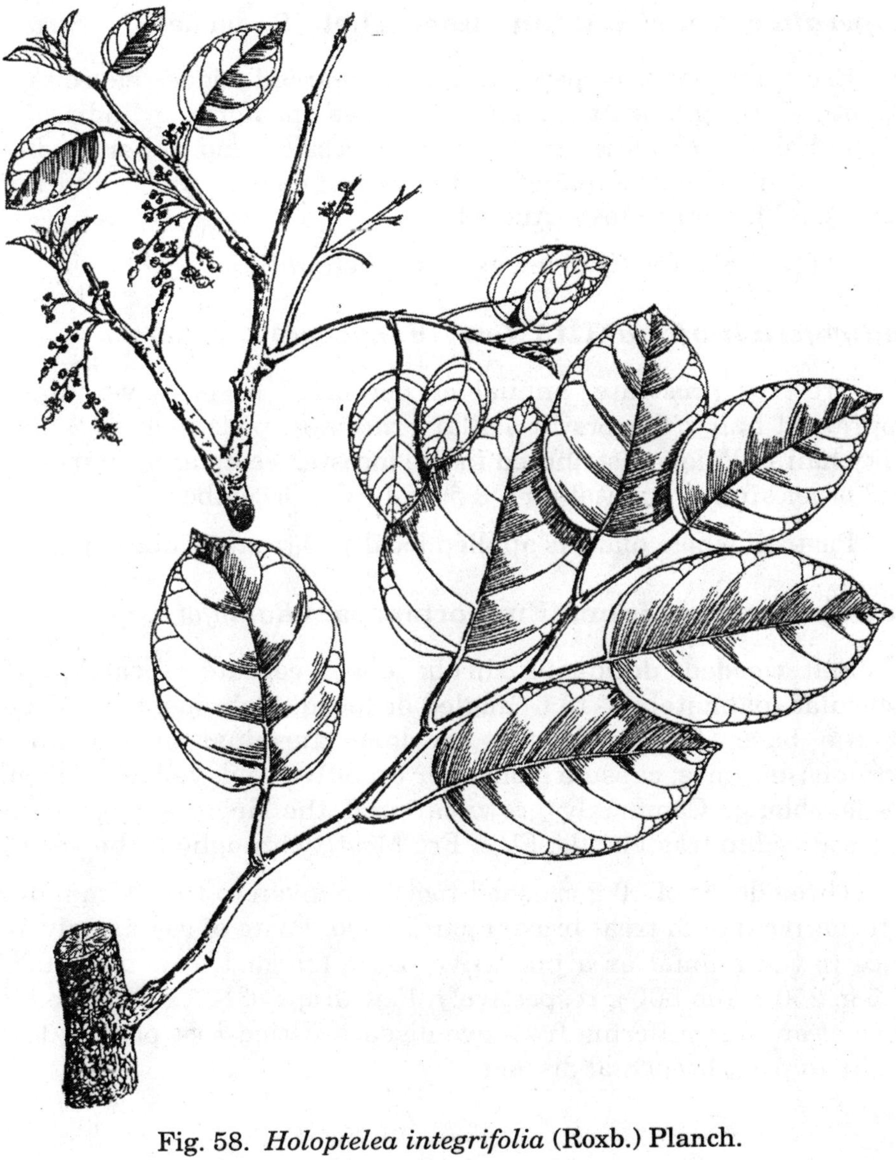

Fig. 58. *Holoptelea integrifolia* (Roxb.) Planch.

Hygrophila auriculata (Schum.) Heine (Acanthaceae)

Hispid annual, herb with thickened nodes; leaves sessile, oblong or lanceolate, hispid in verticels of six at a node; spines axillary; flowers in each axillary whorl; capsule linear - oblong, 4 - 8 seeded. Abundant in swampy habitats, waste places along ditches and canals in association with grasses and sedges. Fl. & Fr.: August – February.

Decoction of 100 g leaves is given orally to animal to treat foot and mouth disease.

Imperata cylindrica (Linn.) Raeuschel. (Poaceae) *Siru*

Erect, rhizomatous perennial, with bearded nodes; leaves tapering at both ends, villous at the base; panicles spiciform, cylindrical, silky white hairy; spikelets in pairs, one sessile and other pedicelled, arranged in racemose panicles. Fairly common in moist and marshy habitats. Fl. & Fr.: May – August.

Decoction of root is given as an anthelmintic.

Indigofera linifolia (L.f.) Retz. (Fabaceae) *Jaljamni*

Erect or prostrate, annual or perennial herb; leaves apiculate, appressed hairy; flowers in axillary racemes; pods globose, apiculate, silky hairs. Widely distributed in the forests, wastelands, parks, lawns and other similar habitats. Fl. & Fr.: July – December.

Paste of whole plant is applied locally to treat wound and sore.

Jatropha curcas Linn. (Euphorbiaceae) *Ratanjot*

Soft wooded, deciduous shrub; leaves cordate - ovate to nearly orbicular, palmately 3- to 5- angled or lobed, glabrous, 5- to 7- nerved at the base; flowers in 6-8 cm long, terminal or extra-axillary corymbose cymes; capsule globose or broadly ovoid, yellow and smooth; seeds oblong. Commonly grown around the fields for fencing, also naturalized in wastelands. Fl. & Fr.: Mostly throughout the year.

Three doses of 10 g crushed roots are given to the animal once on alternative day to treat broken joint/ bone. Paste of roots is given only once to the animal as a purgative. Dose for goat, cow and buffalo is 125 g, 250 g and 500 g respectively. Few drops of latex is poured in the eyes of animal suffering from eye disease. Dried root powder is given orally to treat bronchial disease.

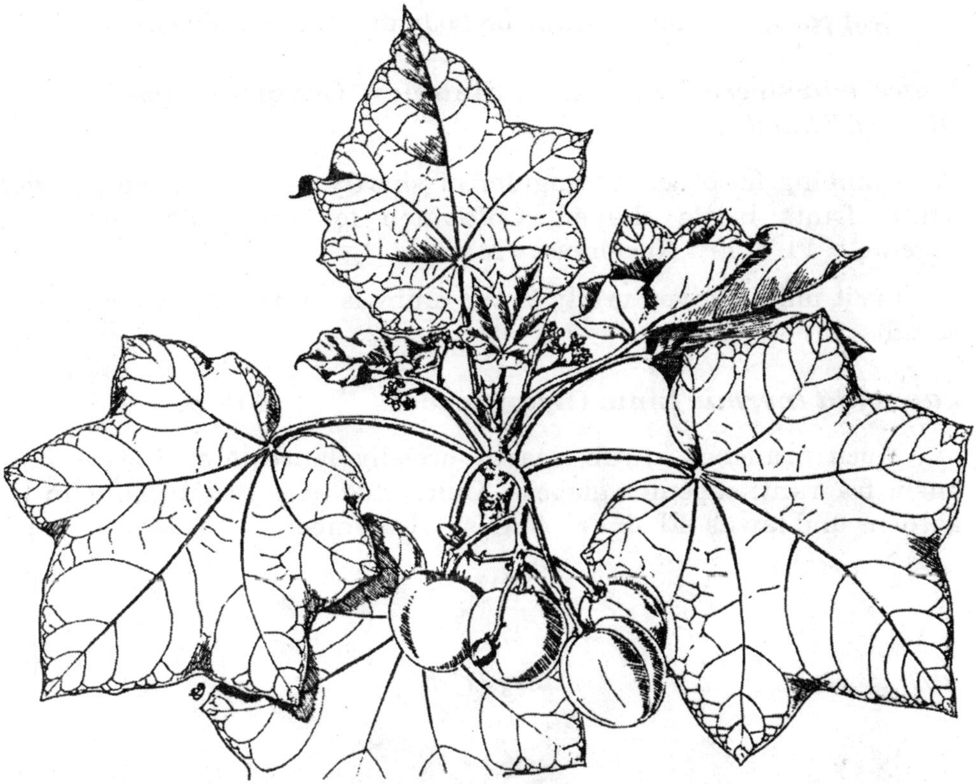

Fig. 59. *Jatropha curcas* Linn.

***Jatropha gossypifolia* Linn. (Euphorbiaceae)** *Ratanjot*

Tall, erect, glandular hairy shrub, with deep reddish - purple branches; leaves orbicular to obovate, palmately 3 to 5 - lobed; flowers in terminal, trichotomous cymes. Naturalized in wastelands near habitations, also cultivated in the gardens and on the edges of fields. Fl. & Fr.: Almost throughout the year.

About 30 – 40 seeds of *Jatropha gossypifolia* are given to animal to treat constipation. Extract of stem is given orally to the animal to treat fractured bone. The decoction of roots is given to domestic animals through drenching tube to treat uterus diseases.

***Kalanchoe pinnata* (Lam.) Pers. (Crassulaceae)** *Patharchata*

Erect, glabrous herb, upto 1 m high; stem obtusely 4 - angled, purple spotted; lower and uppermost leaves simple; middle ones pinnately 3- to 5- foliolate; flowers pendulous in lax panicles. Grow wild in shaded places and along water courses; usually cultivated for ornamental purpose. Fl. & Fr.: December - June.

Leaf paste is applied locally on body to treat skin diseases.

***Lagenaria siceraria* (Molina) Standley (Cucurbitaceae)**
Dhodka, Thumbo, Thumba

Climbing herb; leaves angular or shortly 3- lobed leaves; flowers white; fruits bottle shaped. Cultivated for the fruits cooked as vegetable. Fl. & Fr.: November – March.

Fruit pulp is given orally to the animals to increase the secretion of milk.

***Lawsonia inermis* Linn. (Lythraceae)** *Mahendi*

Much branched shrub; leaves broadly lanceolate; flowers creamish, fragrant; capsules globose. Cultivated as a hedge plant in the gardens and lawns. Fl. & Fr.: August – December.

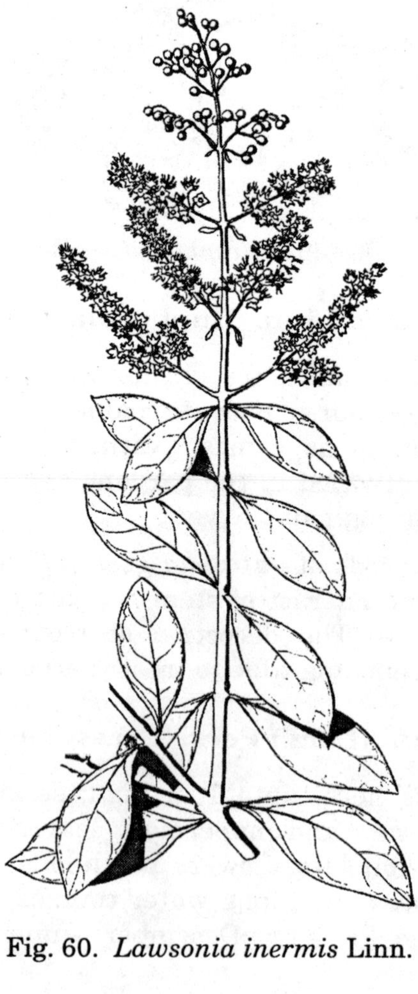

Fig. 60. *Lawsonia inermis* Linn.

Paste of leaves is applied on skin to treat burns. Fresh leaf paste is applied to treat fractured bones and also applied locally to treat foot and mouth disease.

Leea macrophylla **Roxb. ex Hornem. (Leeaceae)** *Dalavad, Lal patti*

Erect herb; with simple, broadly ovate to subcordate leaves; flowers small white; fruits of the size of a small cherry, black, succulent. Rare, in the forest of Southern part of the state. Fl. & Fr.: August – November.

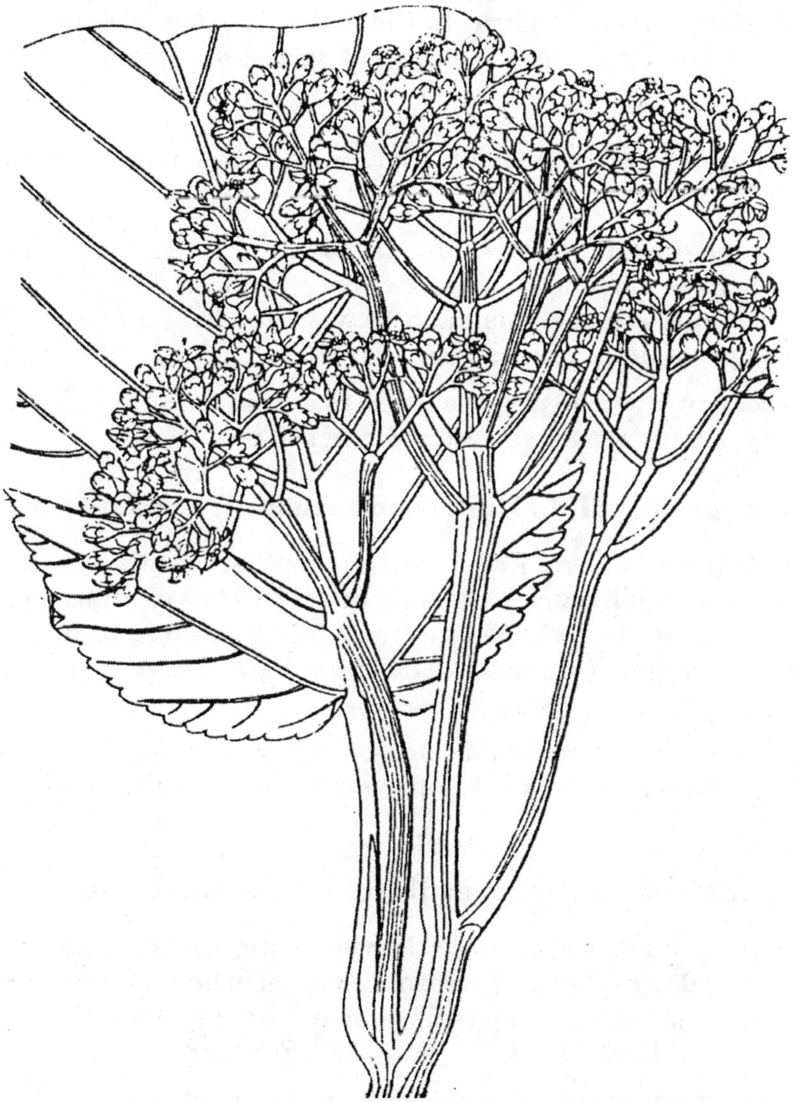

Fig. 61. *Leea macrophylla* Roxb. ex Hornem.

Decoction of 2.5 cm tuber is given to animal through drenching tube to treat food poisoning. Root powder is given orally to treat dysentery. Leaf paste is applied locally to treat fractured bone.

***Leptadenia pyrotechnica* (Forssk.) Decne. (Asclepiadaceae)**
Kheep

Bushy shrub; with caducous, linear - lanceolate leaves; greenish yellow flowers; follicles terete, tapering to a slender beak. Abundantly found on sand dunes, frequently throughout in sandy plains. Fl. & Fr.: August – January.

Infusion of stem is given to the camel to treat flatulence. Tender shoots are cut into small pieces and mixed with fodder for oestrus induction.

***Leptadenia reticulata* (Retz.) Wt. & Arn. (Asclepiadaceae)**
Jhunka

Twining shrub; leaves broadly ovate - lanceolate; flowers in lateral, many - flowered umbellate cyme; follicles broadly lanceolate, with thick curved beak. Common in wastelands and open forests and on the edges of fields and gardens. Fl. & Fr.:Throughout the year.

Decoction of whole plant is given to animal once in a day upto four to five days to increases the secretion of milk.

***Leucas aspera* (Willd.) Link (Lamiaceae)** *Piyari, Kaddiyo*

Densely hairy herb; linear - oblong leaves; flowers sessile or so, in terminal and axillary whorls reaching 2.5 cm in diameter; bracts linear, acute, bristle - shaped; nutlets oblong, smooth, brown. Common from plains to hills throughout the state. Fl. & Fr.: Almost throughout the year.

Bolus prepared from mixture of 10g *Piper longum* (Choti pipli) and 20g whole plant of *Leucas aspera* is given to the animal to treat fever.

***Leucas cephalotes* (Koen. ex Roth) Spr. (Lamiaceae)** *Kubi*

Erect, annual, hispid herb; leaves ovate, subacute, membranous; flowers sessile, in dense, globose, terminal whorls; nutlets obovoid - oblong, rounded at apex, smooth, brown. Common weed in wastelands and cultivated fields. Fl. & Fr.: August – February.

Whole plant is fed to sheep for overall improvement in health.

Lindernia crustacea **(Linn.) F. Muell. (Scrophulariaceae)** *Chotibui*

Diffusely branched, annual herbs, with 4 – angled stem hairy on the angles; leaves ovate; flowers axillary, solitary and subracemose; capsule long, obovate, apiculate. Common from plains to the hills in wet habitats, particularly in the east of Aravalli. Fl. & Fr.: August – February.

Paste of 5-10 g leaves of *Lindernia crustacea* is applied twice in a day to treat eczema.

Luffa acutangula **(Linn.) Roxb. (Cucurbitaceae)** *Jangli taroie*

Extensive, scabrous climber; leaves 10-20 by 10-20 cm, palmately 5- to 7- angled or lobbed; flowers yellow to pale yellow; fruits 15-30 by 5 - 10 cm, not warty; seeds 10-12 by 6-8 mm, ovate, compressed, black. Naturalized in wastelands, outskirts of forest, on the boundaries of gardens and field among hedges. Fl. & Fr.: July – October.

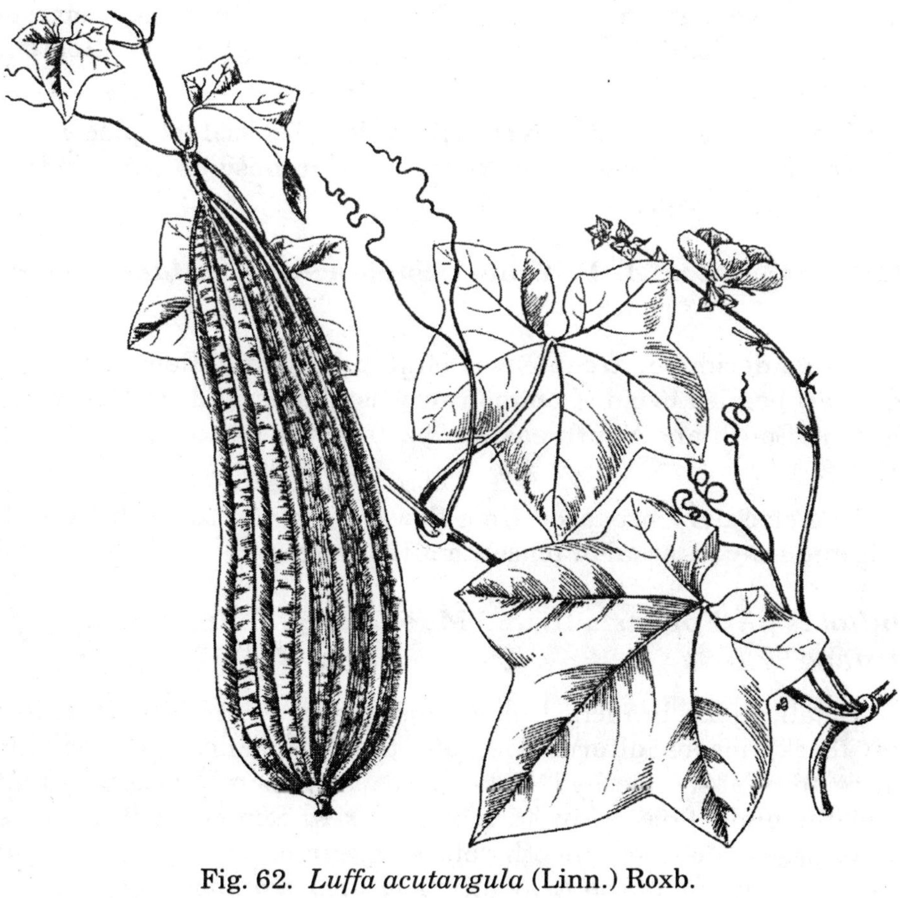

Fig. 62. *Luffa acutangula* (Linn.) Roxb.

Decoction prepared from the mixture of fruits of *Luffa acutangula*, seeds of *Trachyspermum ammi* and black salt is given to the animal by drenching tube to treat flatulence. The powder of whole plant is mixed with curd and given orally upto three days to treat the disease locally known as *'Pannichera'* (diarrhoea and dysentery) and *'Mottichera'* (vomiting).

Luffa echinata **Roxb. (Cucurbitaceae)** *Jangli turi, Kakora*

Climber; tendrils bifid; leaves reniform – orbicular; flowers white; fruits ovoid, bristly. Common on the outskirts of forests and along the fences of gardens and fields. Fl. & Fr.: August – October.

Fruit of *Luffa echinata* is crushed and mixed in musturd oil. This mixture is given to domestic animal to treat stomach disorder.

Lycium barbarum **Linn. (Solanaceae)** *Mureli, Arak – mehendi*

Spinous shrubs, with solitary or fascicled, oblong-lanceolate leaves. Flowers creamish-white. Fruits red when ripe. Common in scrub forests, particularly in desertic zones. Fl. & Fr.: September-February.

Decoction of root is given orally for disposal of placenta after delivery. A snuff of powdered root is given in nose of horse to treat in respiratory diseases.

Madhuca indica **J. F. Gmel. (Sapotaceae)** *Mahua, Mahuwa, Mauo*

Large deciduous tree; leaves elliptic - obovate; flowers in axillary fascicles; berries ovoid. Common in wastelands and on the fringes of forest in South and South eastern parts of the state. Fl. & Fr.: March – June.

The electuary prepared from flowers is given to animals orally to facilitate easy disposal of placenta after delivery.

Mallotus philippensis **(Lam.) Muell. - Arg. (Euphorbiaceae)** *Sindhur*

Small, much branched, dioecious, evergreen tree, with thin dark grey bark; leaves alternate, ovate to ovate lanceolate, acuminate, entire to slightly toothed, subcoriaceous, puberulous and glandular beneath; male flowers in terminal spikes, female solitary in short spike; seeds globose, smooth, black. Common in the dry deciduous forests in the east of the Aravalli. Fl. & Fr.:December – March.

Red powder extracted from the capsule of this plant is poured on cotton and tied on the broken horns of animals to stop bleeding and for early healing.

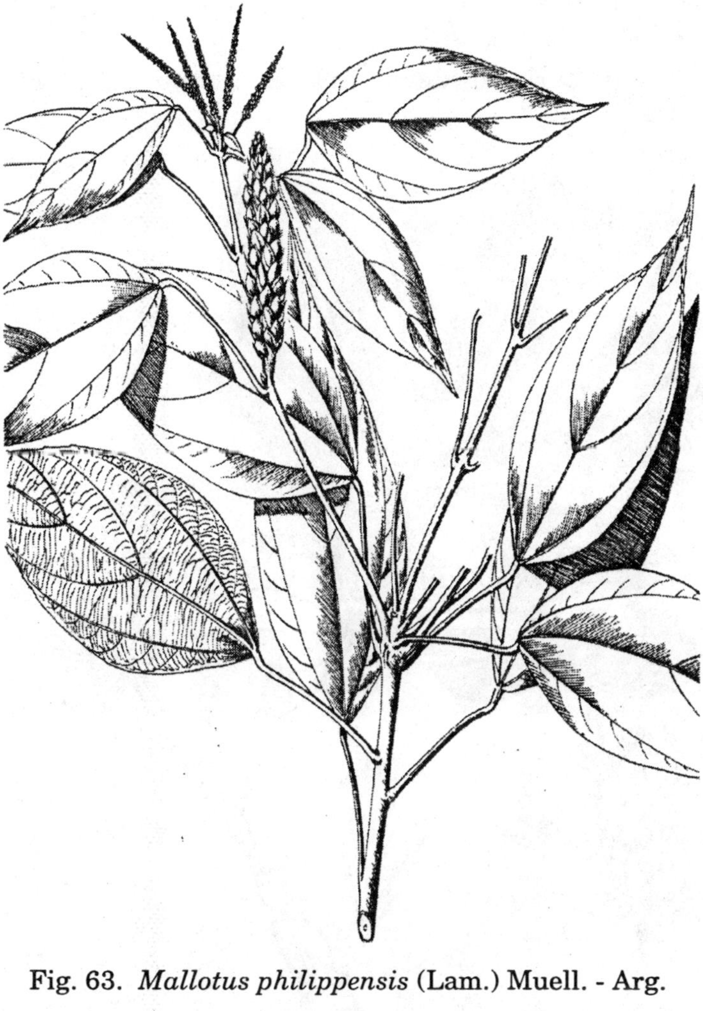

Fig. 63. *Mallotus philippensis* (Lam.) Muell. - Arg.

Mangifera indica **Linn. (Anacardiaceae)** *Amba, Amboo, Aam*

Evergreen tree; leaves oblong - lanceolate; flowers polygamous in panicles; drupes yellow when ripe. Indigenous in South-east Rajasthan; also planted in the orchards. Fl. & Fr.: December – July.

Decoction of 50 g bark is given to the animal by drenching tube to treat diarrhoea. 200 g bark is crushed and boiled with 1 kg barley and 1 kg jaggery and after cooling given orally two times in a day in morning and evening to increase the secretion of milk. About 100 g bark is crushed and fed with jaggery to bulls to increase sexual power.

Manilkara hexandra **(Roxb.) Dub. (Sapotaceae)** *Chotta runkhdi*

Evergreen tree, with deeply furrowed bark; leaves elliptic - obovate or oblong; flower in axillary fascicles of 2 -6; berries ovoid, 1 - seeded. Fl. & Fr.: October – April.

Paste of stem bark powder is applied in the throat of animal to treat tonsillitis.

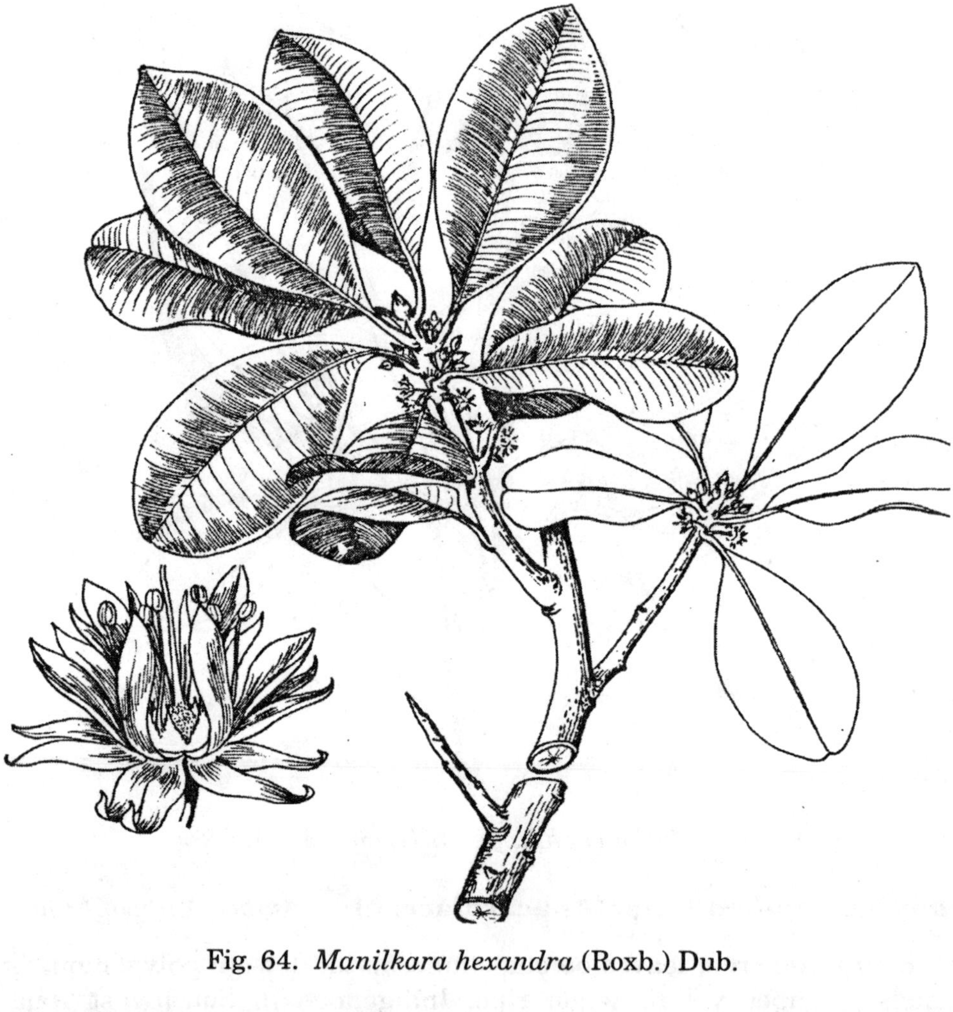

Fig. 64. *Manilkara hexandra* (Roxb.) Dub.

Martynia annua **Linn. (Martyniaceae)** *Kagala, Bichhu – kanto* (Plate 7)

Glandular pubescent herb; stem fistular; leaves ovate-cordate, drooping; fruits woody, beetle-shaped, hooked at the tip. Naturalized along roads, railway-lines and fringes of forests. Fl. & Fr.:August – October.

Decoction of whole plant is applied locally on the wound of animal as an antiseptic. Paste of stem bark is applied locally to treat bone fracture.

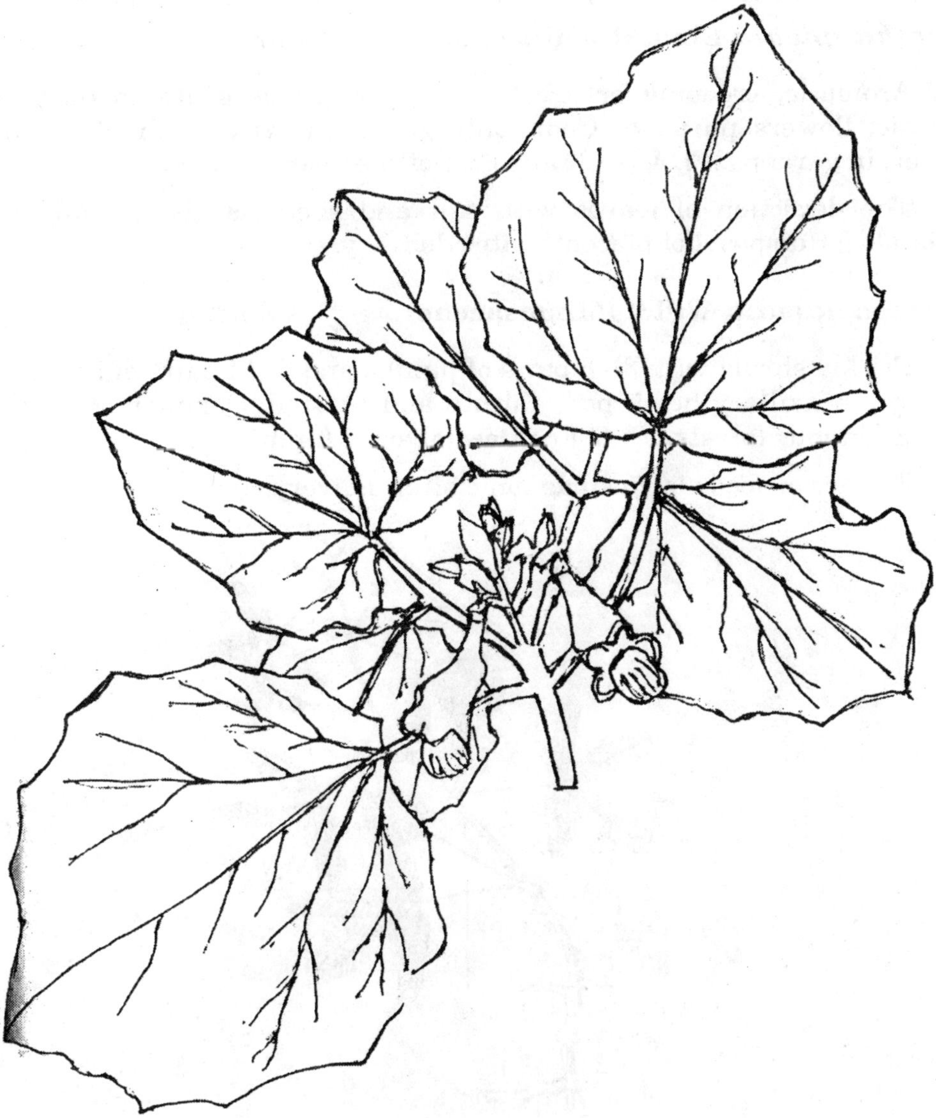

Fig. 65. *Martynia annua* Linn.

Melia azedarach **Linn. (Meliaceae)** *Bakain, Desi - neem*

Tree; leaves 1 to 3 - pinnate; flowers in axillary panicles; drupes ellipsoid - oblong, 4 to 5- seeded. Rarely found in wastelands; usually planted along the roads. Fl. & Fr.: Nearly throughout the year.

About 25-30 g leaves of *Melia azedarach* is given to the animal once in a day upto 3 days for removal of internal parasites. Excess quantity is poisonous.

Mentha spicata Linn. (Lamiaceae) *Pudina*

Aromatic, creeping or ascending herb; leaves ovate to ovate - elliptic; flowers purplish. Commonly grown in areas with plenty of water, in gardens. Fl. & Fr.: Most part of the year.

The decoction of leaves with salt and sugar is given orally to animals for disposal of placenta after delivery.

Mimosa hamata Willd. (Mimosaceae) *Amado*

Prickly shrub; with 3 - 6 pairs of pinnae and 5- 14 pairs of leaflets; flowers in axillary head; pods falcate and twisted. Common in scrub and deciduous forests. Fl. & Fr.: December – March.

Powder of seeds is given as tonic after delivery.

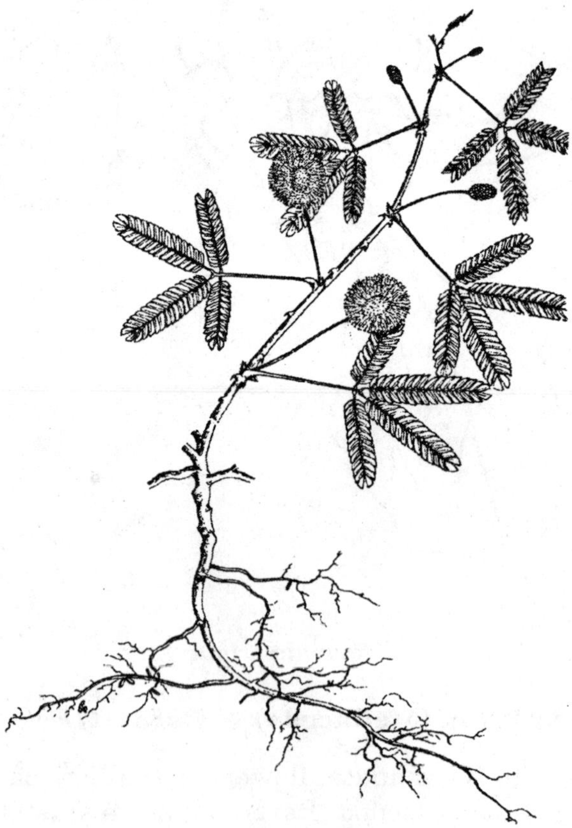

Fig. 66. *Mimosa pudica* Linn.

***Mimosa pudica* Linn. (Mimosaceae)** *Chuimuai*

Much branched, prickly herb; pinnae sensitive, 2-4 pairs; flowers in globose heads; pods flat, slightly curved. Often found as an escape in the gardens; usually cultivated. Fl. & Fr.: September – November.

Root extract is given to animal especially oxen suffering from neck tumour due to continuous yoke ploughing. After giving extract for three days, rest is given for about six days to ox for complete recovery.

***Mirabilis jalapa* Linn. (Nyctaginaceae)** *Gulabbas*

Erect, glabrescent to pubescent herb, with tuberous roots; leaves ovate, acuminate or acute subentire, glabrescent, under surface with rahpides; flowers subsessile, in fascicles, scarlet, showy; nut subglobose. Naturalized as a weed in cultivated fields. Fl. & Fr.: Almost throughout the year.

Root decoction is applied locally to treat wound.

***Moringa oleifera* Lam. (Moringaceae)** *Sainjna*

Small tree, bark corky, wood soft; with 3-pinnate leaves, pinnae and pinnules opposite, deciduous; flowers in spreading axillary panicles; pods long, 9-ribbed; seeds 3- angled, the angles winged. Planted in gardens. Fl. & Fr.: Throughout the year.

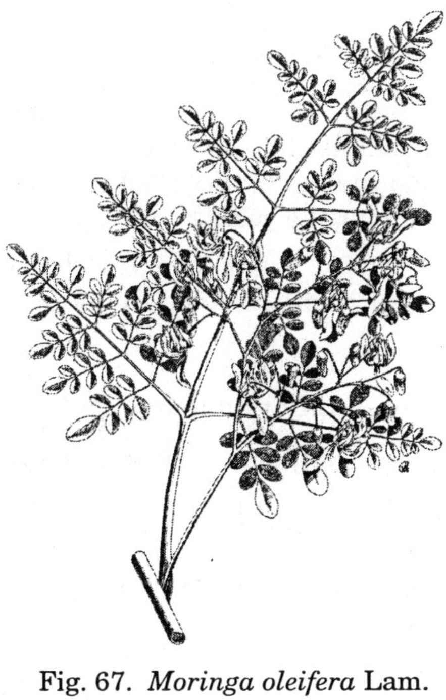

Fig. 67. *Moringa oleifera* Lam.

Paste of leaves and stem bark is given with sugar to increase lactation. Decoction of leaves is given orally to treat swelling, boils and anthrax.

***Momordica dioica* Roxb. ex Willd. (Cucurbitaceae)**
Jangli karela, Kikora

Perennial climber, with tuberous roots; leaves ovate, mucronate, entire or 3 to 5 - lobed; flowers yellow; fruits ellipsoid or ovoid, beaked, densely echinate, with soft spines. Common on the hedges of cultivated fields, gardens and outskirts of forest. Fl. & Fr.: August – October.

Extract of tuber is applied externally on skin of animal to kill ectoparasites.

***Mucuna pruriens* (Linn.) DC. (Fabaceae)** *Kamach, Konch*

Twining, hirsute, annual herb; leaves trifoliate; flowers 2-3 cm long in drooping, 6-30 flowered raceme; pods slightly curved at both ends in opposite directions, densely bristly. Common in wastelands and open forests among the clumps of trees and shrubs. Fl. & Fr.: August – April.

One or two pods of *Mucuna pruriens* are mixed with jaggery (*Saccharum officinarum*) or wheat bread and fed to the female animal twice a day for five days for oestrus induction.

***Musa paradisiaca* Linn. (Musaceae)** *Kela, Kell*

Tree like, stoloniferous herbs; leaves spirally arranged oblong; flowers yellow, lower female, upper male in drooping spathaceous spikes; fruits 3- gonous oblong. Cultivated in the orchards for edible fruits. Fl. & Fr.: Throughout the year.

Fresh leaves are fed to the cow after delivery for disposal of placenta. Fruits mixed with milk are fed to animal to treat swelling of udder and mastitis.

***Nerium oleander* Linn. (Apocynaceae)** *Kaner*

Evergreen shrub; leaves linear – elliptic; flowers white or red in cymes. Cultivated for ornamental purposes. Fl. & Fr.: Throughout the year.

Root paste is applied on infected part of body to treat eczema.

Nicotiana tabacum **Linn. (Solanaceae)** *Tambakhu*

Glandular-pubescent herbs, with pinkish flowers and ovate capsules. Cultivated in the garden.

Fl. & Fr.: Most part of the year.

Leaf paste is applied locally to treat foot diseases. Mixture of 10 g dried leaves of tobacco; 50 g Sodium carbonate and 500 ml mustard oil is given to the animal to treat flatulence.

Nyctanthes arbor -tristis **Linn. (Oleaceae)** *Har-singar* (Plate 7)

Large shrub, 4 - angled branches; leaves opposite, ovate or ovate - lanceolate; flowers white to orange, fragrant, sessile, 3- to 5- together on axillary, solitary or fascicled peduncles; capsule orbicular, compressed. Abundant in the forests; also cultivated in the gardens for ornamental purpose. Fl. & Fr.: August – November.

About 50 ml extract of leaves is mixed with water and given to animal through drenching tube twice in a day to treat colic.

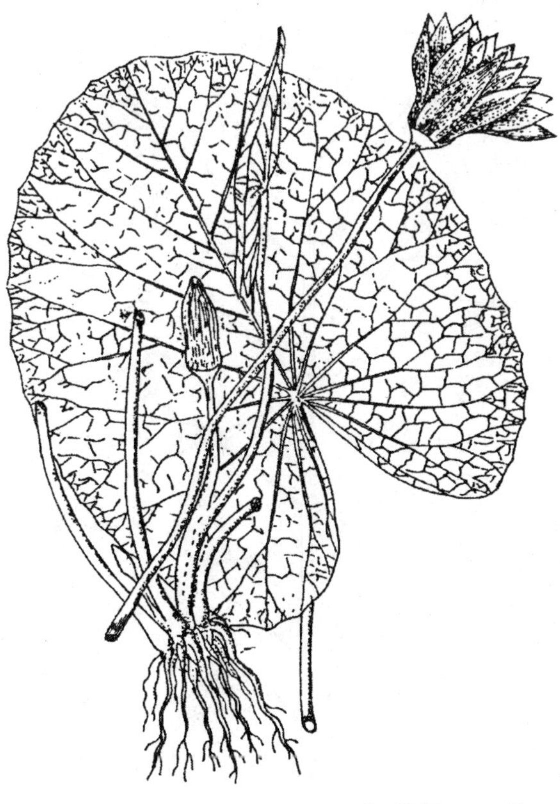

Fig. 68. *Nymphaea nauchali* Burm. f.

Nymphaea nauchali **Burm. f. (Nymphaeaceae)** *Kamal*

Perennial, aquatic herb; leaves 8 -20 cm in diameter, orbicular or elliptic - sagittate, when young peltate; flowers solitary; fruits globose; seeds longitudinally striate. Common in ponds, ditches and tanks. Fl. & Fr.: August – February.

About 100 ml rhizome extract is mixed with curd and given orally four – five times in a day to treat diarrhoea.

Ocimum americanum **Sims. (Lamiaceae)** *Tulsi, Ban - tulsi, Jangli tulsi*

Annual herb; ovate - lanceolate to ovate - oblong leaves; flower whorls in long racemes, white; nutlets ovoid. Common weed in open wastelands; sometimes cultivated. Fl. & Fr.: Almost throughout the year.

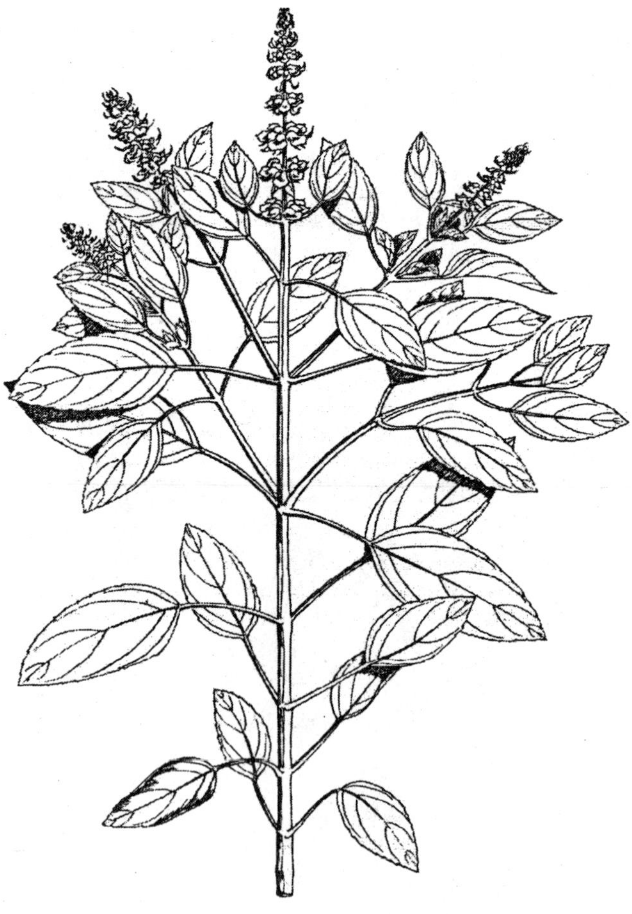

Fig. 69. *Ocimum americanum* Sims.

Paste of 50 g fruits of *Amygdalus communis*, 50 g *'lac'*, 10 g seeds of *Foeniculum vulgare*, 10 g whole plant of *Ocimum americanum* is given to the animal with fodder to treat leucorrhoea. 200 g seed powder is mixed with 250 g milk fat, 500 g wheat flour and 500 g jaggery. Laddoos (local sweet) of 150 g thus prepared are given orally once in a day for one month to treat tuberculosis or asthmatic attack in animals.

***Ocimum tenuiflorum* Linn. (Lamiaceae)** *Tulsi*

Perennial herb or undershrub; with ovate-lanceolate or ovate-oblong leaves; flowers white, whorled in long raceme; nutlets ovoid. Common in wastelands; also cultivated. Fl. & Fr.: October - January.

Mixture of paste of 20 leaves of *Ocimum tenuiflorum*, 20 ml honey and 50 ml urine of a calf is given to the animal orally to treat cancer. This treatment results in weight gain and good health of animal. Paste of about 10 g leaves of *Ocimum indicum* is applied on the skin to treat scabies.

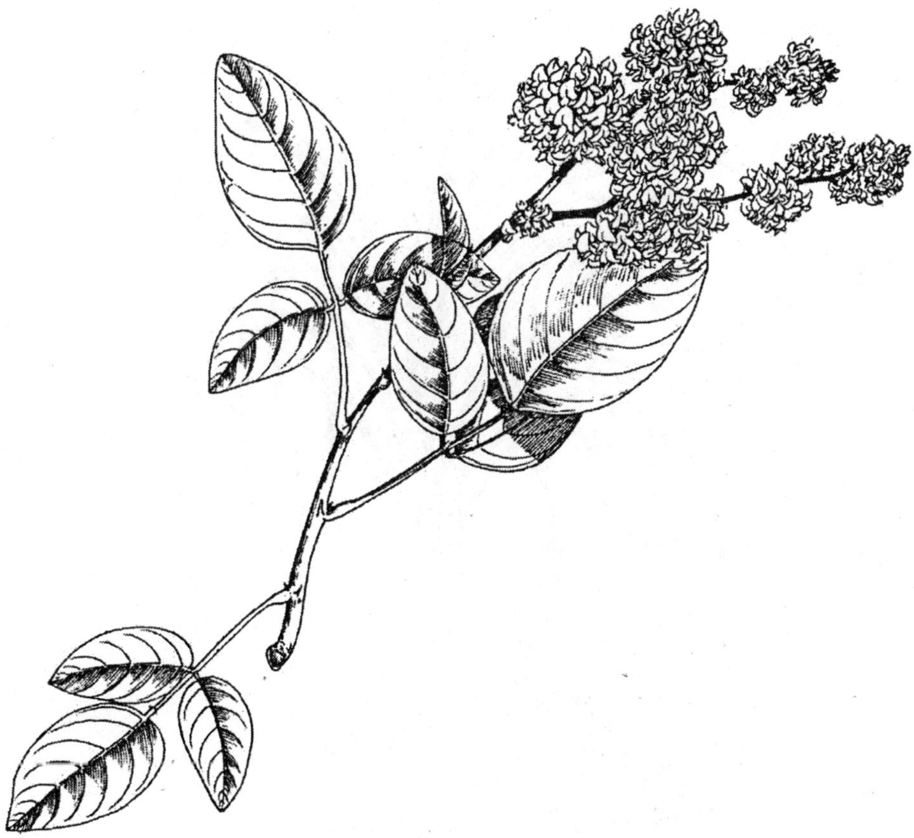

Fig. 70. *Ougeinia oojeinensis* (Roxb.) Hochr.

Ougeinia oojeinensis **(Roxb.) Hochr. (Fabaceae)** *Sandan, Tanas*

Deciduous tree; leaves 3- foliolate; flowers in short, fascicled racemes arising from the nodes of old branches, white; pods flat. Rare, in the wasteland. Fl. & Fr.: March – May.

Decoction of bark is poured on hooves of the animal to treat painful infections. The bark decoction is also given to treat dysentery.

Pandanus fascicularis **Lam. (Pandanaceae)** *Kewra* (Plate 7)

Much branched, thick bush or small tree, with aerial roots; leaves drooping, spirally arranged ensiform, with recurved marginal spines; spathes very sweet scented; drupes pyramidal woody. Rare, along the streams in the forests. Fl. & Fr.: April – July.

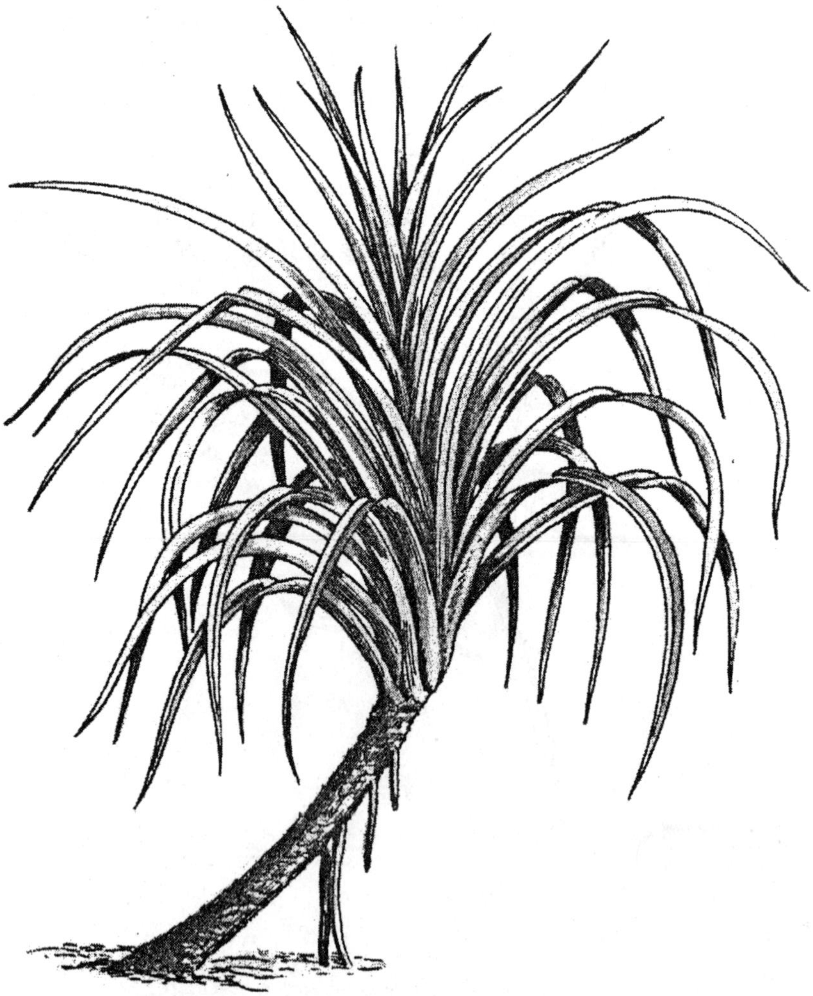

Fig. 71. *Pandanus fascicularis* Lam.

About 250 ml of root extract is given with water to bulls, oxes and bullocks to increase sexual power. Root extract is given orally to treat prolapsed of uterus.

***Panicum miliaceum* Linn. (Poaceae)** *Hamali*

Tufted, tall annual, 50 - 150 cm high, leaves linear - lanceolate, often covered with tubercle - based hairs; ligule a narrow ciliate rim; panicle long lax. Often found as a weed in irrigated fields. Fl. & Fr.: August – October.

Either grains or whole plant is given to the animal to increase secretion of milk.

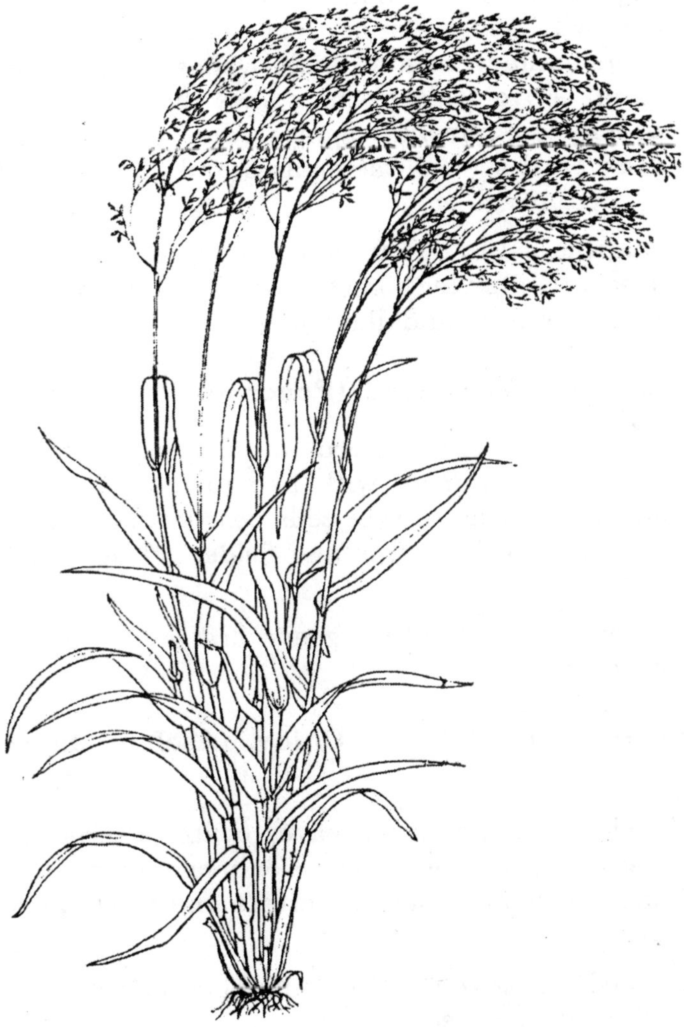

Fig. 72. *Panicum miliaceum* Linn.

Parkinsonia aculeata **Linn. (Caesalpiniaceae)** *Parkinsonia*

Large shrubs or small trees, armed, glabrous; leaves bipinnate; rachis short and ending into a spine; leaflets 25-30 pairs, 0.4-0.5 cm long, ovate-oblong; flowers sub-axillary racemes, bright yellow; pods linear, constricted between the seeds, glabrous; seeds oblong, smooth, mottled. Naturalized in wastelands, also cultivated for ornamental purposes. Fl. & Fr.: March-June.

Paste of leaves is given orally to goat to treat constipation.

Pedalium murex **Linn. (Pedaliaceae)** *Dakhni-gokhru* (Plate 8)

Glandular pubescent annual herb; stems and branches often slightly rough with scaly glands; leaves obovate – oblong, repand-dentate; flowers axillary, solitary, pale- yellow; fruits narrowed at the base, pyramidal – ovoid above the spines, bluntly 4 – angled, with stout sharp conical horizontal spines from the angles. Frequently occur on sandy hard soil in wasteplaces and along road sides. Fl. & Fr.: August – December.

Whole plant is fed to the animal as it cools body in summers.The plant is dipped in water for sometime and this water is given to the animal to treat dysentery and diarrhoea.

Pennisetum typhoides **Burm.f. (Poaceae)** *Bajaro*

Tall, robust annuals, with terminal long panicles with villous or woolly rachis; each involucre with two to many spikelets; lemmas pubescent on the margins; anther-cells bearded. A very common rainy season crop cultivated for grains and fodder. Fl. & Fr.: September – December.

Boiled grains mixed with jaggery are given to the animal to induce labour pain.

Pergularia daemia **(Forssk.) Chiov. (Asclepiadaceae)** *Manda-bheti*

Hispid twining undershrub; leaves ovate, acuminate; flowers in drooping lateral corymbose cymes. Common among bushes on the edges of fields, gardens, fringes of forests and wastelands. Fl. & Fr.: March – December.

Crushed pods are given to the animal for oestrus induction and to treat foot and mouth disease.

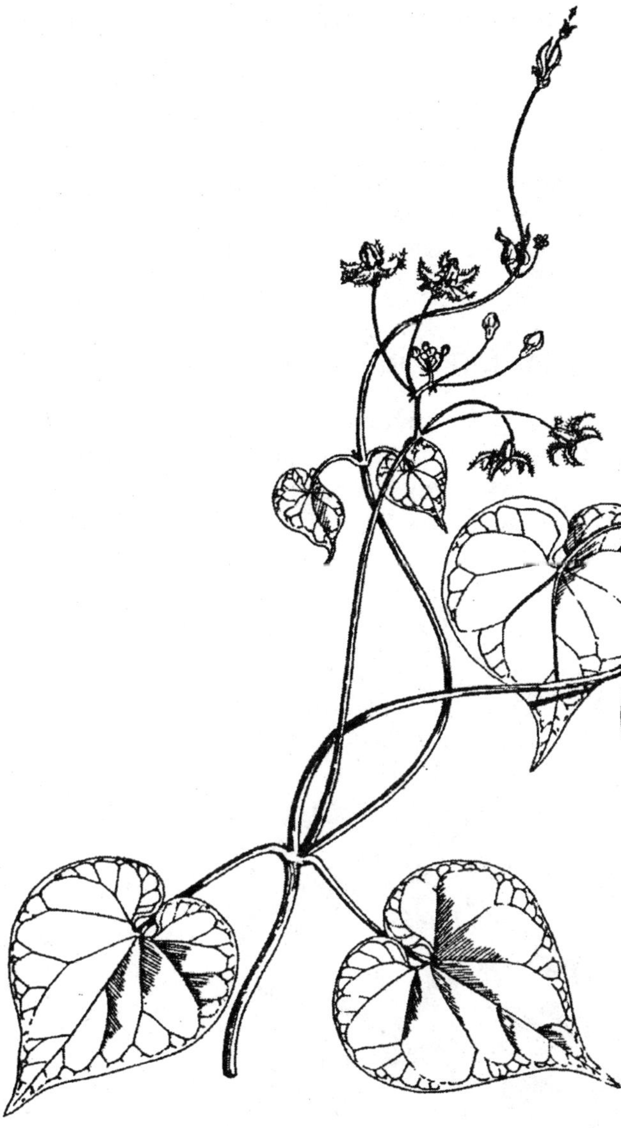

Fig. 73. *Pergularia daemia* (Forssk.) Chiov.

***Phaseolus mungo* Linn. (Fabaceae)** *Urad*

Trailing, hispid herb, with 3 - foliolate leaves and yellow flowers; pods linear, turgid. Cultivated as a rainy season pulse crop. Fl. & Fr.: August – October.

The animal is fed with bread made up of *Phaseolus mungo* flour mixed with seed oil of *Sesamum indicum* to treat foot and mouth disease.

Phoenix sylvestris **(Linn.) Roxb. (Arecaceae)** *Khajoor, Tar, Teri, Khajoori*

Tall, unbranched, monoecious, graceful palm, with straight or crooked trunk; leaves pinnate; inflorescence a spadix; spathes woody, scurfy, separating into boat-shaped valves; drupes scattered; seeds rounded at both ends, deeply grooved on one side. Common in wastelands; abundant in low lying area. Fl. & Fr.: February – August.

Fruits are given to the animal daily for oestrus induction.

Phyllanthus fraternus **Webst. (Euphorbiaceae)** *Bhui-amla*

Glabrous herb; with closely distichous, leaves oblong, resembling a compound leaf; flowers yellowish - green, hidden under the leaves; disc of female flowers irregularly cup - shaped with 6 - 9 segments. Weed in cultivated fields and gardens. Fl. & Fr.: August – December.

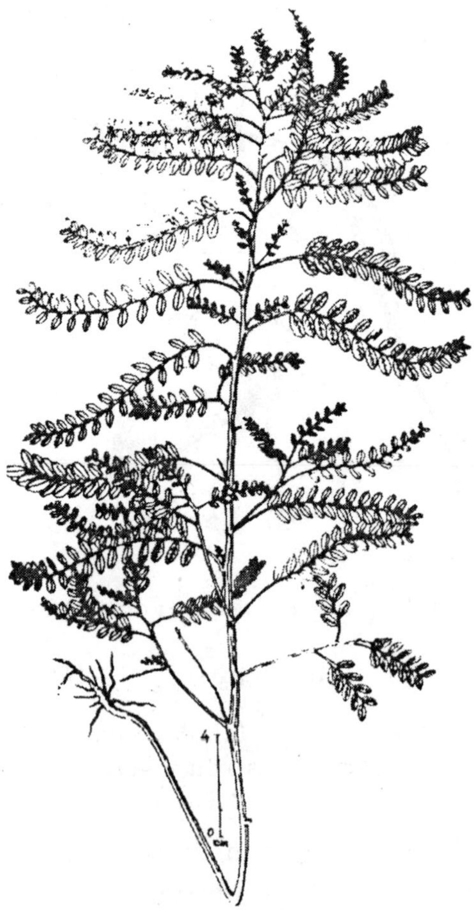

Fig. 74. *Phyllanthus fraternus* Webst.

About 10 g leaves are fed to the animal with fodder once in a day upto two-three days to treat fever. Ash of 250 g leaves is mixed with 100 ml oil of *Pongamia pinnata* and applied locally to treat septicemia.

***Phyllanthus virgatus* Forst. f. (Euphorbiaceae)** *Bhui–amla, Dudhi*

Erect or decumbent - ascending, annual - perennial herb; with woody base; leaves elliptic - lanceolate to oblong; flowers pedicelled, axillary, solitary, unisexual. Weed in cultivated fields, grasslands and gardens. Fl. & Fr.: August – December.

About 10 g leaves are given to the animal with fodder once in a day for two-three days to treat fever.

***Piper betel* Linn. (Piperaceae)** *Nagarbel, Pan*

Perennial climber; leaves cordate; flowers in catkin inflorescence. This species is not found wild, often cultivated in Rajasthan at very low scale. Fl. & Fr.: September – April.

About 20 leaves are fed to the animal with fodder to treat flatulence. Leaf decoction is given orally in fever.

***Pithecellobium dulce* (Roxb.) Benth. (Mimosaceae)** *Jangal - jalebi, Kikar*

Medium-sized tree, armed with spines; pinnae and leaflets one pair each; flower heads dirty white; pods circinate or twisted. Planted on the edges of gardens. Fl. & Fr.: March – August.

Paste of stem bark is applied locally to treat swelling.

***Peperomia pellucida* Linn. (Peperomiaceae)** *Pipramul*

Perennial climber; leaves cordate; flowers white in catkin inflorescence. Rare, found in moist places of hilly forests. Fl. & Fr.: September - April.

About 150 g seeds of *Piper nigrum* are mixed with 280 g milk fat and given daily upto 3 days to treat mastitis. During this treatment oily and acidic foodstuffs are not given to the animal.

***Plumbago zeylanica* Linn. (Plumbaginaceae)** *Chitrak, Chitraval* (Plate 8)

Erect or straggling undershrub; leaves ovate-lanceolate or oblong, acute, contracted at the base into a petiole; flowers white, in axillary and terminal, 5-30 cm long racemes combined into leafy panicles; capsule furrowed, enclosed within the persistent calyx. Common in wastelands and open forests among bushes. Fl. & Fr.: Most part of the year.

Decoction of two to four leaves of *Plumbago zeylanica* and 250 g seeds of *Trachyspermum ammi* (*'Ajwain'*) is given to the animal to treat indigestion and flatulence.

Polygonum plebeium **R. Br. (Polygonaceae)** *Lalbuti*

Diffusely branched, prostrate herb; leaves oblong or oblanceolate-linear; flowers sessile, almost concealed by stipules; nutlets rhomboid - trigonous. Abundant in drying ponds along the roads, bank of rivers and tanks. Fl. & Fr.: July – November.

About 50 g decoction of whole plant is given orally upto five days for secretion of more milk. Plant ash with mustard oil is applied locally to treat eczema.

Pongamia pinnata **(Linn.) Pierre (Fabaceae)** *Karanj, Kavja, Safed chitrak*

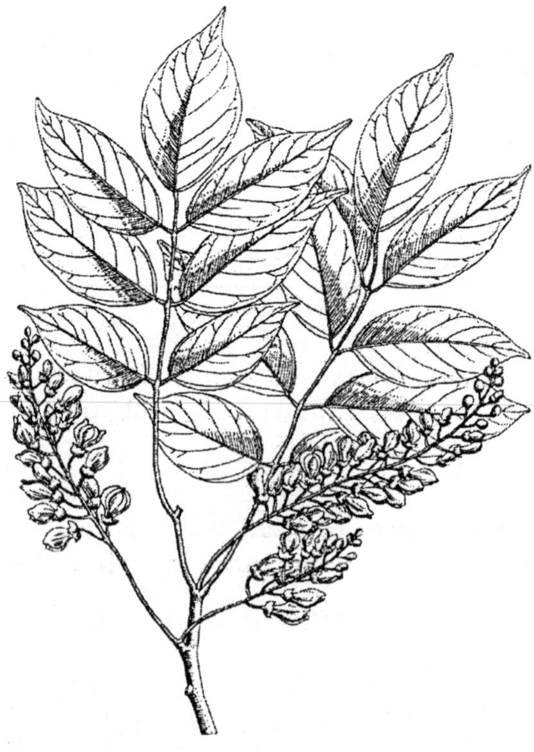

Fig. 75. *Pongamia pinnata* (Linn.) Pierre

Tree, 7-10 m high with greyish bark; leaves imparipinnate; leaflets 5-9, elliptic or ovate -oblong; flowers in fascicles of 2 - 4 on the rachis of axillary racemes; pods obliquely oblong, woody, glabrous, not winged. Common in wastelands, along roads. Fl. & Fr.: March – June.

Seed oil is used to treat skin disease of domestic animals. Seed oil with leaf paste of *Adhatoda zeylanica* is applied as balm on hump sore of cows and buffaloes. Extract of the bark is given to buffalo-calves when they drink too much milk.

***Portulaca oleracea* Linn. (Portulacaceae)** *Kungan*

Prostrate or diffuse herb; leaves succulent, obovate-spathulate; flowers yellow; capsules obovoid. Common weed in fields, gardens and other moist grounds, like river bed. Fl. & Fr.: August - December.

Decoction of whole plant is given orally in fever.

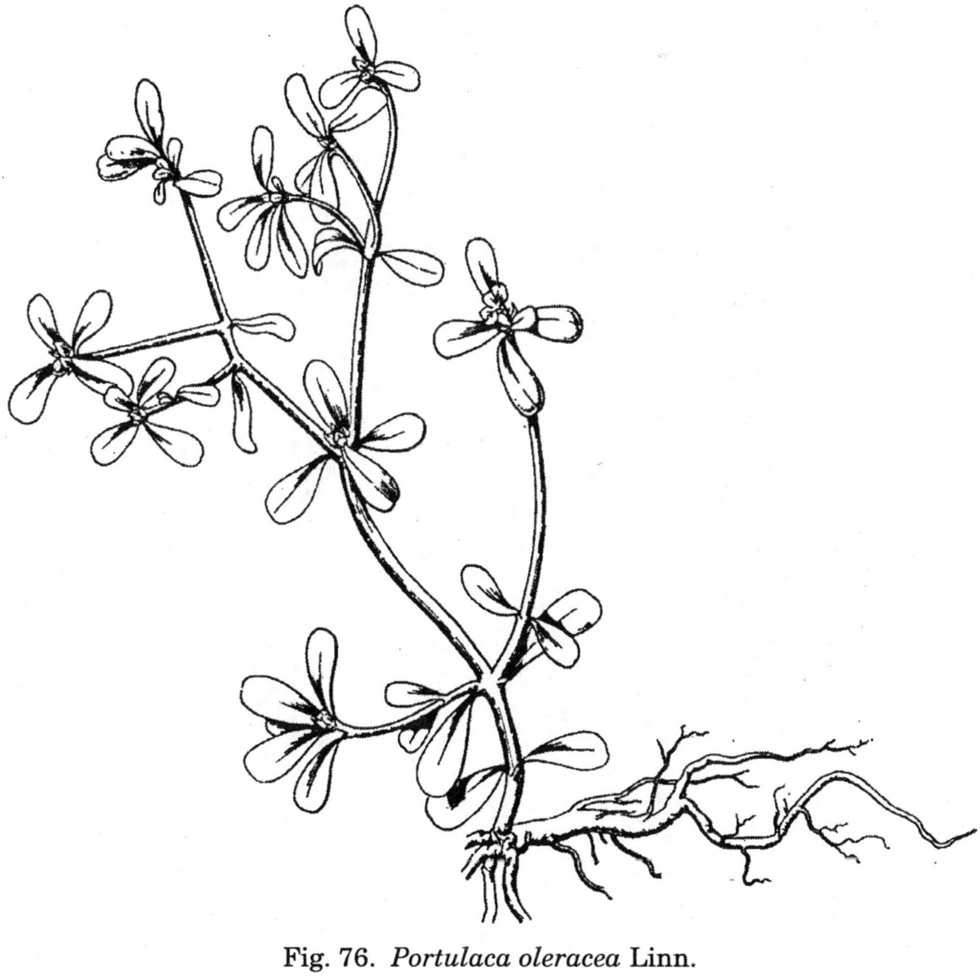

Fig. 76. *Portulaca oleracea* Linn.

***Prosopis cineraria* (Linn.) Druce (Mimosaceae)** *Khejri, Sangri, Khejda, Janti.*

Medium sized tree; bark grey, rough with deep fissures or cracks; leaves 2-pinnate; flowers yellow; pods pendulous slender, pointed at the apex; seeds oblong to suborbicular. Abundantly found throughout the Shekhawati region but rare in hilly terrain. Fl. & Fr.: March - July; rarely in November – December.

Leaf is fed with fodder to treat mouth ulcer.

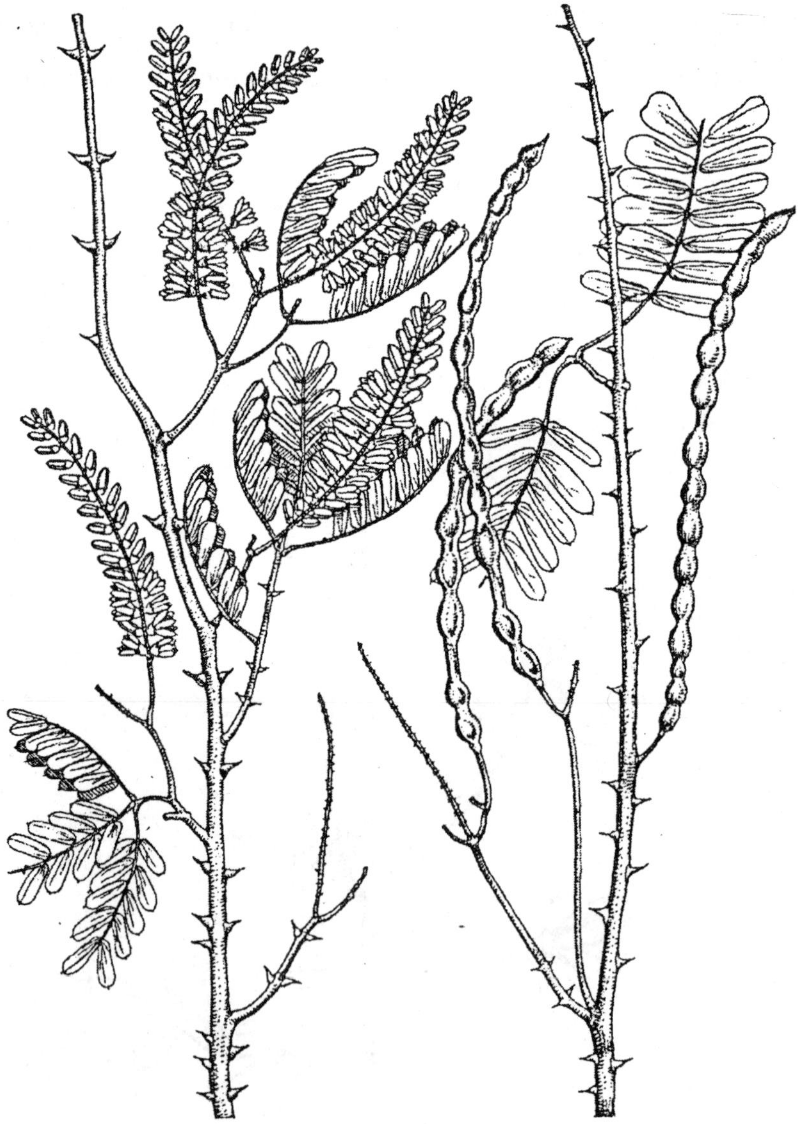

Fig. 77. *Prosopis cineraria* (Linn.) Druce

***Prosopis juliflora* (Swartz) DC. (Mimosaceae)** *Kikar, Zeri-bavar*

Small trees or shrubs, armed with axillary spines; pinnae 1-2 pairs, leaflets 15-25 pairs; spikes pale-yellow, pendulous; pods sub-falcate, subcompressed. Common in wastelands. Fl. & Fr.: Most part of the year.

Crushed leaves are applied on wounds.

***Pterocarpus marsupium* Roxb. (Fabaceae)** *Bijasal*

Deciduous tree, with crooked stem and spreading branches; leaves elliptic or ovate; flowers pale yellow in fusco-paniculate racemes; pods suborbicular, winged, glabrous. Rare in mixed deciduous forests. Fl. & Fr.: April – June.

200 g decoction of stem bark is given orally to treat dysentery.

***Pueraria tuberosa* (Roxb. ex Willd.) DC. (Fabaceae)** *Vidarikand*

Woody twiner; with 3 leaflets; flowers bluish, in axillary racemes; pods bristly, constricted between the seeds. Rare, in wastelands among the clumps of trees and shrubs. Fl. & Fr.: July – October.

Boiled tubers are fed to the animal after delivery for providing nutritious diet.

***Pupalia atropurpurea* Moq. (Amaranthaceae)** *Sihitti*

Annual or biennial herb; leaves, ovate or elliptic – lanceolate, acuminate, mucronate, suddenly contracted at the base; flowers in lax pedunculate terminal spikes; utricles ovoid, membranous; seeds oblong – ellipsoid, with subtruncate ends. Common in gravelly to rocky habitats in wastelands, open forests, edges of field etc.among bushes. Fl. & Fr.: Most part of the year.

Paste of 30 g roots is given orally, twice in a day only for one day to treat infection in anus as well as on tail.

***Rhus mysurensis* G. Don (Anacardiaceae)** *Dansaria*

Armed shrub or small tree; with 3- foliolate, coarsely serrate leaves; flowers polygamous in panicles; drupes subglobose. Common in scrub forests on the Aravalli Fl. & Fr.: July - October.

Leaf paste of *Rhus mysurensis* is applied on the body to treat allergy / rashes / eczema.

***Ricinus communis* Linn. (Euphorbiaceae)** *Arandi*

Large, erect shrub with fistular stem and glaucous-grey or reddish, smooth bark; leaves 10-30 cm in diameter, palmately 5 to 10 lobed; flowers in pyramidal panicle; capsule globose, spiny of 3 cocci; seeds oblong - ovoid, smooth, shining, mottled, caruncled. Naturalized in wastelands near habitation. Fl. & Fr.: Almost throughout the year.

About 200 ml seed oil is given orally to the animal to treat indigestion, fever and flatulence. About 100 ml seed-oil is also given orally one or two times in a day to treat constipation.

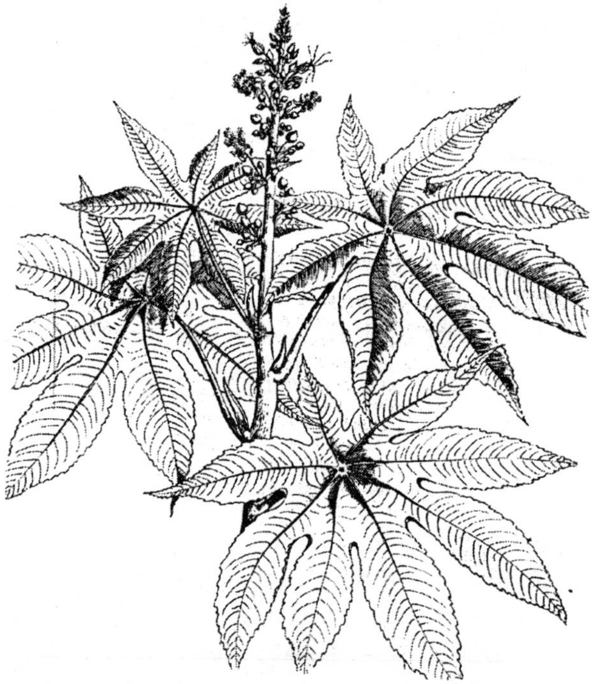

Fig. 78. *Ricinus communis* Linn.

***Saccharum officinarum* Linn. (Poaceae)** *Ganna, Hantha*

Tall, perennial, rhizomatous plant, with juicy culms; leaves wide and laminated right to the base; spikelets awnless, glumes glabrous. Cultivated mainly in south and south-eastern parts of Rajasthan for culm-juice which is used for making jaggery. Fl. & Fr.: January onwards.

Jaggery (*Saccharum officinarum*) and human fallen hairs are wrapped over an iron rod warmed and applied on the wound to stop bleeding instantly. About seven to eight kg sugarcane is fed to the animal for disposal of placenta after delivery.

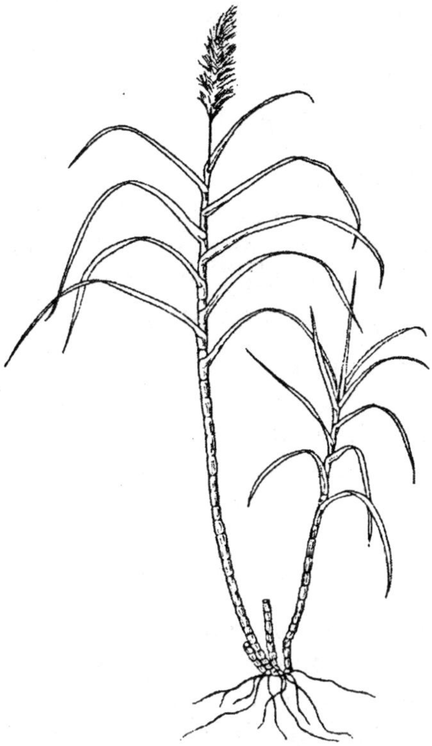

Fig. 79. *Saccharum officinarum* Linn.

Salvadora oleoides **Decne. (Salvadoraceae)** *Jaal, Pilu*

Evergreen small tree with soft whitish yellow wood; twisted trunk and drooping branches, trunk bark blackish-grey; leaves linear-lanceolate; flowers sessile, greenish - white; fruits drupe, globose, yellow when ripe. Common in saline and sandy habitat. Fl. & Fr.: December – March.

The paste prepared with ash of whole plant with milk is applied locally to treat scabies of camel. Leaf extract is applied locally to treat wound and mastitis.

Salvia aegyptiaca **Linn. (Lamiaceae)** *Hingot*

Much - branched, straggling under-shrub; branches divaricate rigid, hairy; leaves subsessile, linear-lanceolate, acute, crenate, much wrinkled, nerves prominent; flowers - whorls 2 to 4 flowered, borne in long raceme; nutlets oblong-ellipsoid, smooth, bluish - black. Common in moist places, along road - sides, borders of cultivated fields and in scrub forests. Fl. & Fr.: December- March.

Powder of dried seeds is given orally with drenching tube to treat diarrhoea.

Sarcostemma viminale **(Linn.) R.Br. (Asclepiadaceae)** *Khir, Khimp* (Plate 8)

Branched, leafless, succulent, straggling shrub; stem pubescent when young; flowers greenish white, in sessile terminal umbel; follicles solitary, tapering at both ends. Common on rocky habitat in the hilly tract. Fl. & Fr.: August – November.

Decoction of whole plant is given to the animal through drenching tube twice in a day upto 7 days to treat rheumatism. Extract of whole plant is given to the animal to treat digestive disorders. Infusion of whole plant is applied by the rural people on wound of dog and snake bite.

Sesamum indicum **Linn. (Pedaliaceae)** *Kala - til*

Erect, glandular- pubescent annual with angular, sulcate stem; leaves elliptic-lanceolate, upper entire, lower 2 to 3- segmented; flowers axillary, solitary; capsule oblong-quadrangular; seeds black or white. Truly naturalized wild from plains to the hills. Fl. & Fr.: August – November.

200 g seed oil is given orally to the animal to treat foot and mouth disease. Leaf extract is given to cows and goats to treat disease locally known as '*Matoti*'. Seed oil (250 g) is given orally to domestic animals to treat foot and mouth disease.

Sesbania aculeata **(Willd.) Pers (Fabaceae)** *Solehut*

Erect, weak-stemmed, annual herbs or undershrubs, 1.0-2.5 m high; leaflets 12-50 pairs, 0.5-1.5 by 0.2-0.5 cm, linear-oblong, mucronate, glabrous, stipellate; flowers in axillary, 3 to 6 flowered recems, yellow; pods 20-30 cm long, linear, subterete, tomentose, beaked, glabrous. Common in rice fields and other swampy places. Fl. & Fr.: August – Ocober.

Seeds are given with fodder to bring the animal in heat. About 50 ml root extract is given orally to the animal to treat intestinal worms.

Shorea robusta **Gaertn. f. (Dipterocarpaceae)** *Sal*

Trees usually large, bark gray to dark reddish brown, fissured, flaky; stipules fugacious, lanceolate, small; petiole 2-2.5 cm, buff scabrous-pubescent; leaf blade 10-40 by 5-24 cm, ovate to oblong, thinly leathery; flowers subsessile, on panicles; fruit sepals unequal, spatulate, sparsely pubescent. Cultivated mainly for its wood. Fl. & Fr.: Febuary – July.

About 250 g leaves are given to the animal with fodder to treat nematodal infection. Decoction of roots is given to treat typhoid and fever.

***Sida ovata* Forssk. (Malvaceae)** *Khariti, Barath, Dabe, Bal*

Stellately hispid, 170 cm high, under shrub; leaves stipulate, linear, 4 mm long, tomentose; petioles 1.1 cm long; lamina base truncate, 4.2 by 4.0 cm, palmately 5- veined, stellately-tomentose, obtuse; axillary, solitary flowers; mericarps 7- 8, 2 awned. Common in plains and rare in hilly tracts. Fl. & Fr.: November – January.

Whole plant is fed to animal with fodder to treat bodyache. Smoke of burning seeds is employed to remove the worms of teeth.

***Solanum virginianum* Linn. (Solanaceae)** *Ringni Bhor-rigani*

Sparsely pubescent, divaricately branched herb; with ovate – oblong leaves; flowers white globose; yellow red or purple fruits. Common weed in cultivated field during winters. Fl. & Fr.: November – March.

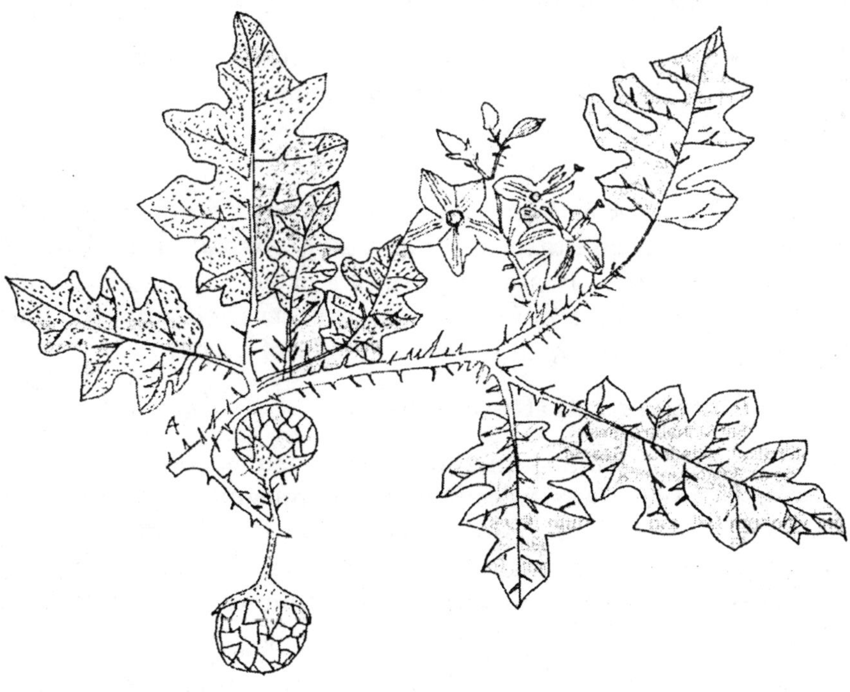

Fig. 80. *Solanum virginianum* Linn.

Smoke of burning seeds is employed to remove the worms of teeth. Seed and leaf extract is applied to treat sores and wounds of animal.

***Sorghum halepense* (Linn.) Pers. (Poaceae)** *Baru*

Stout, erect perennial; with creeping, stoloniferous root-stock; leaves broadly linear- lanceolate, acuminate, base rounded or sub-amplexicaul; panicles lax, open; spikelets 2-nate in pairs. Common in wastelands and in fallow fields. Fl. & Fr.: September- December.

Chapatti made from seed flour of *Sorghum halepense* is given to the animal upto 3 to 5 days to treat diarrhoea and weakness.

***Sorghum vulgare* Linn. (Poaceae)** *Jawar*

Tall robust annual grass; leaves broad with prominent midrib; inflorescence decompound panicle; spikelets large, broad, hairy, two type of spikelets, sessile and stalked, stalked spikelet neuter; sessile spikelet hermaphrodite; fruit caryopsis oblong-globose, white. Cultivated plant. Fl. & Fr.: September – December.

1 kg. alum ($KAl(SO_4)_2.12.H_2O$), one kg. salt and 100 gm grain of *Sorghum vulgare* are mixed and given to the animal for disposal of placenta after delivery.

***Soymida febrifuga* (Roxb.) A. Juss. (Meliaceae)** *Rohina*

Tree; leaves entire, crowded at the end of branches; flower in axillary and terminal panicles; capsules ovoid. Occasionally found in the mixed deciduous forests on the hilly slopes. Fl. & Fr.: February – June.

About 100 g bark of *Butea monosperma* and *Soymida febrifuga* is crushed with 500 ml of butter milk and given to the animal thrice in a day to treat diarrhoea. Paste prepared by crushing 20 g of stem bark and 10 g roots of *Calotropis gigantea* are crushed and the paste is applied on eye and bandaged to treat opacity of cornea.

***Spermacoce stricta* L.f. (Rubiaceae)** *Agio*

Annual herb; stems 4-angled, hispid; leaves opposite or verticillate, linear - lanceolate, acute, revolute-margined; stipules connate with leaf-bases forming a truncate-fimbriate tube; flowers in axillary and terminal; seeds ellipsoid, brown, smooth, with a ventral groove. Abundant in the forests and often in wastelands, particularly in the hilly tracts. Fl. & Fr.: August - December.

Decoction of the plant is given to the animal to treat vulvo-vaginal- uterine prolapse.

***Syzygium cumini* (Linn.) Skeels (Myrtaceae)** *Jamun*

Large trees; leaves 10-14 by 3-6 cm, chartaceous, ovate-lanceolate, obtuse – acuminate; cymes panicled, usually solitary; flowers fragrant, sessile, in short compact or laxly paniculate axillary cymes, pale-geenish-white; corolla calyptrate; berries globose or oblong, purple. Commonly planted as an avenue tree and for its edible fruits; often found in the forests. Fl. & Fr.: February – September.

Paste of 100 g bark is mixed with 500 ml curd or butter milk and this mixture given through drenching tube to the animal to treat diarrhoea.

***Tamarindus indica* Linn. (Caesalpiniaceae)** *Aamli, Imail, Katara, Amlyaum*

Evergreen tree; leaflets 6-12 pairs, linear - oblong, subcoriaceous, glabrous; flowers in lax racemes; pods falcate, linear - oblong, with rough, fibrous, grey epicarp Naturalized in waste places and often in the forests. Also planted in the gardens and along the roads. Fl. & Fr.: November- March.

Pods and leaves mixed with water are fed to animal to treat the stomach pain after eating castor.

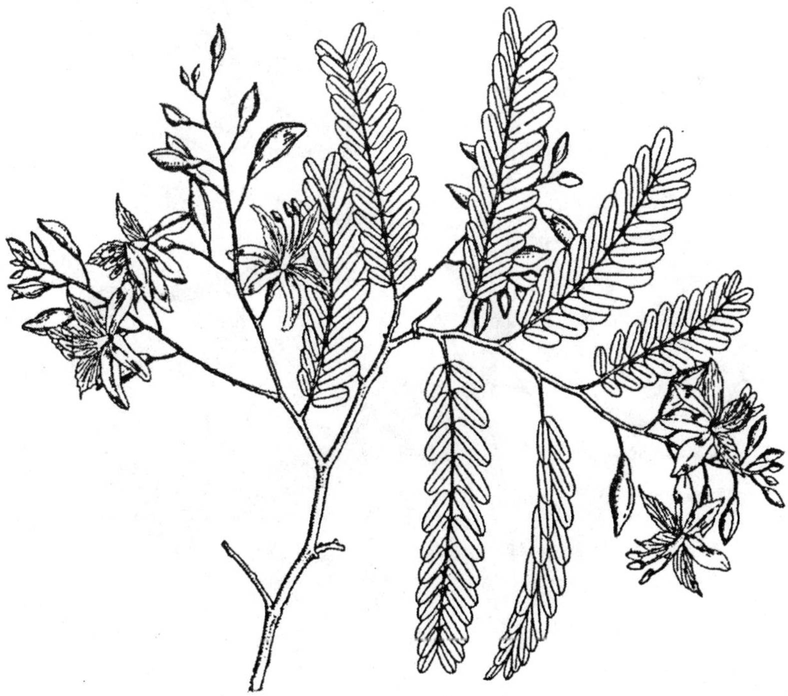

Fig. 81. *Tamarindus indica* Linn.

***Tecomella undulata* (Sm.) Seem. (Bignoniaceae)** *Rohida*

A glaucescent shrub or small tree; stem and branches minutely stellately hairy when young; branches drooping and leaves simple; flowers yellow-orange in terminal racemes or panicles; capsules linear, curved; seeds winged at apex. Commonly found in sandy plains and dunes but very rarely occur on gravelly, clayey, hard soil. Fl. & Fr.: January – May.

Oil is applied locally to treat rashes on skin.

***Tectona grandis* L.f. (Verbenaceae)** *Sagwan, Hagwan, Sag*

Deciduous tree; with broadly elliptic large leaves; flowers terminal, long cymes; drupes subglobose, stellately tomentose. A chief component of deciduous forests, dominating in Southern parts of the state. Fl. & Fr.: August - November.

Paste of leaves is applied twice in a day on the skin to treat eczema and other skin diseases.

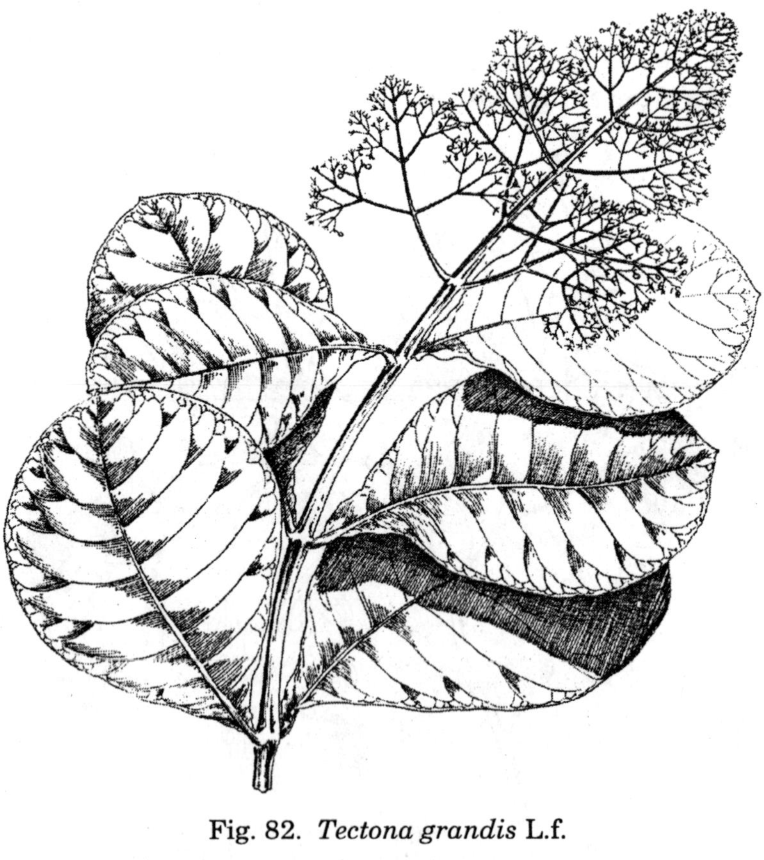

Fig. 82. *Tectona grandis* L.f.

***Tephrosia purpurea* (Linn.) Pers. (Fabaceae)** *Dhamaso*

Perennial, woody herb, with 11-21 leaflets; reddish - purple or bright pink to white flowers in leaf - opposed racemes; pods linear. Gregariously occur on hard clayey or gravelly soils in association with *Capparis decidua, Calotropis procera, Crotalaria burhia, Tephrosia apollinia, Indigofera linnaei, Tribulus terrestris* etc. Fl. & Fr.: July – November.

Roots are fed to animal to treat swelling and rheumatism. Paste prepared by grinding few chillies and red gram (*Cicer arientinum*) to treat constipation.

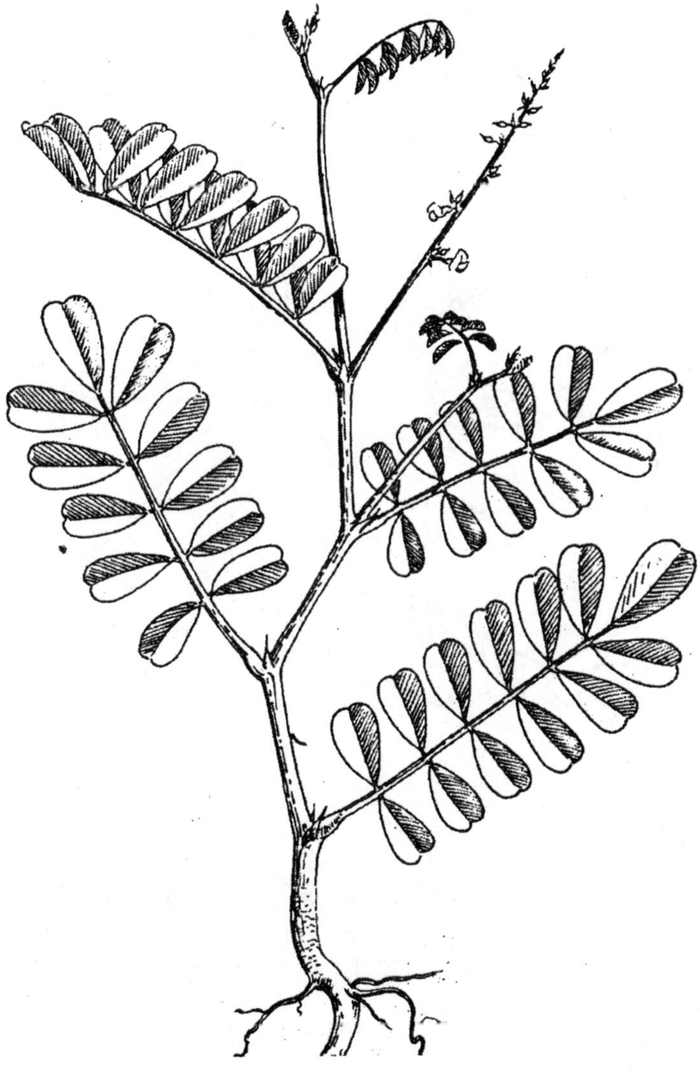

Fig. 83. *Tephrosia purpurea* (Linn.) Pers.

Terminalia arjuna **(Roxb.) Wight and Arn. (Combretaceae)**
Arjun, Kaduaa, Kohda

Trees, with smooth bark; leaves elliptic oblong to suborbicular in axillary spike or terminal panicles; Drupes ovoid to obovoid-oblong. Common in the forests. Fl. & Fr.: March - November

About 300 ml. decoction of bark is given thrice a day for three days to treat body weakness.

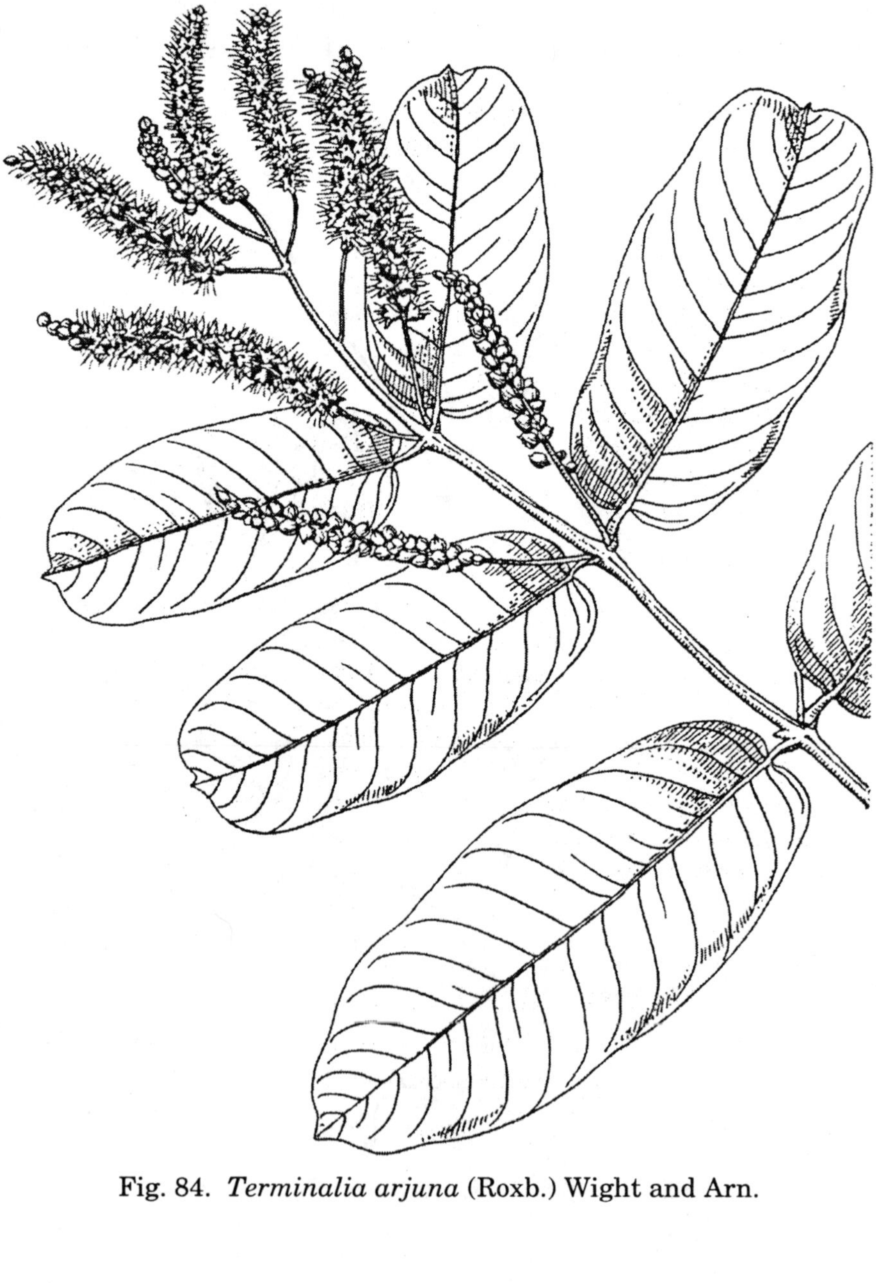

Fig. 84. *Terminalia arjuna* (Roxb.) Wight and Arn.

***Terminalia bellirica* (Gaertn.) Roxb. (Combretaceae)** *Bahera, Veda*

Deciduous tree, 10-30 m high, bark grey, longitudinally fissured; leaves broadly obovate, cuneate, glabrous, coriaceous; flowers in axillary spike; drupes ovoid or ellipsoid, 5-ridged, grey - velvety. Common in mixed deciduous forests. Fl. & Fr.:February - August

Pulp of about 750 g fresh fruits or about 500 g powder of dried fruits is given orally twice in a day upto 7 days to treat diarrhoea.

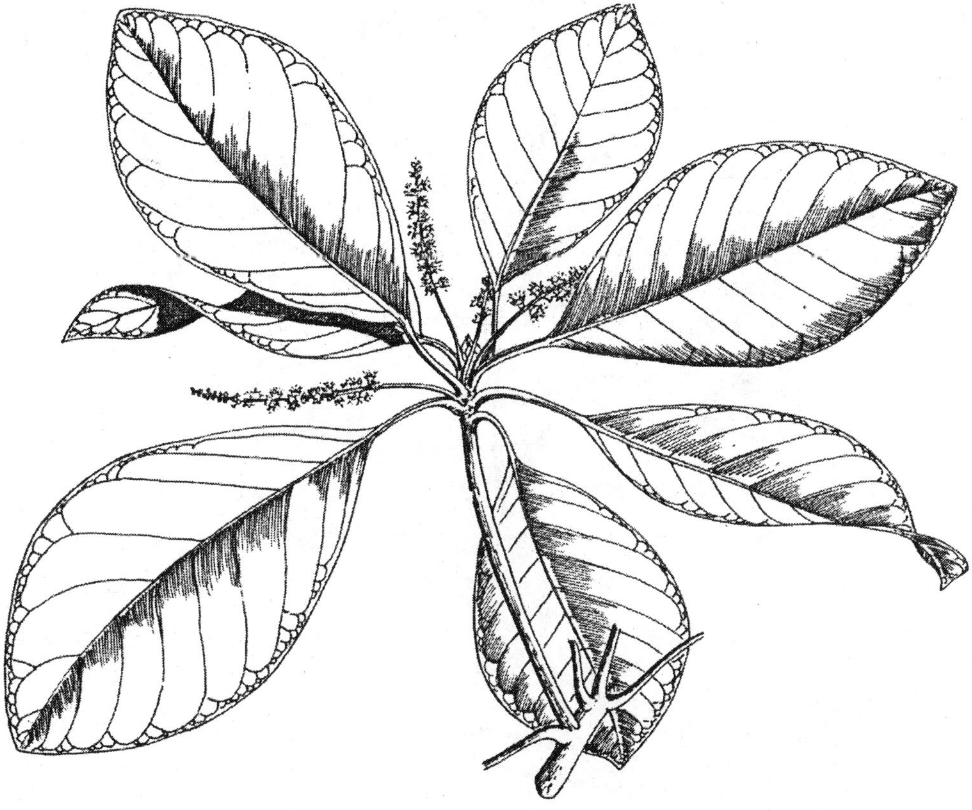

Fig. 85. *Terminalia bellirica* (Gaertn.) Roxb.

***Terminalia chebula* Retz. (Combretaceae)** *Harad*

Large, deciduous trees, 8-20 m high; bark dark brownish-grey, fissured; young parts tomentose. Leaves alternate, long petiolate, 7.5-12.0 by 4.0-10.5 cm, elliptic-oblong or ovate- oblong, rounded at both ends, at length glabrous. Flowers in terminal, panicled spikes, white or pale yellow. Fruits 2.5-4.0 by 1.5-2.5 cm, ovoid, ellipsoid or ellipsoid-obovate, glabrous. Rare, found in dry deciduous forests and wastelands. Fl. & Fr.: March – November.

About 50 g fruits of *Terminalia chebula*, 50 g rock salt, 50 g seeds of *Trachyspermum ammi*, 25 g seeds of *Cuminum cyminum*, 25 g *Elytraria cardamomum* (chhoti ilaychi), 50 g sodium bicarbonate and 500 g jaggery are mixed and bolus of 150g of this mixture is given orally for three days to treat gastro-intestinal disorders.

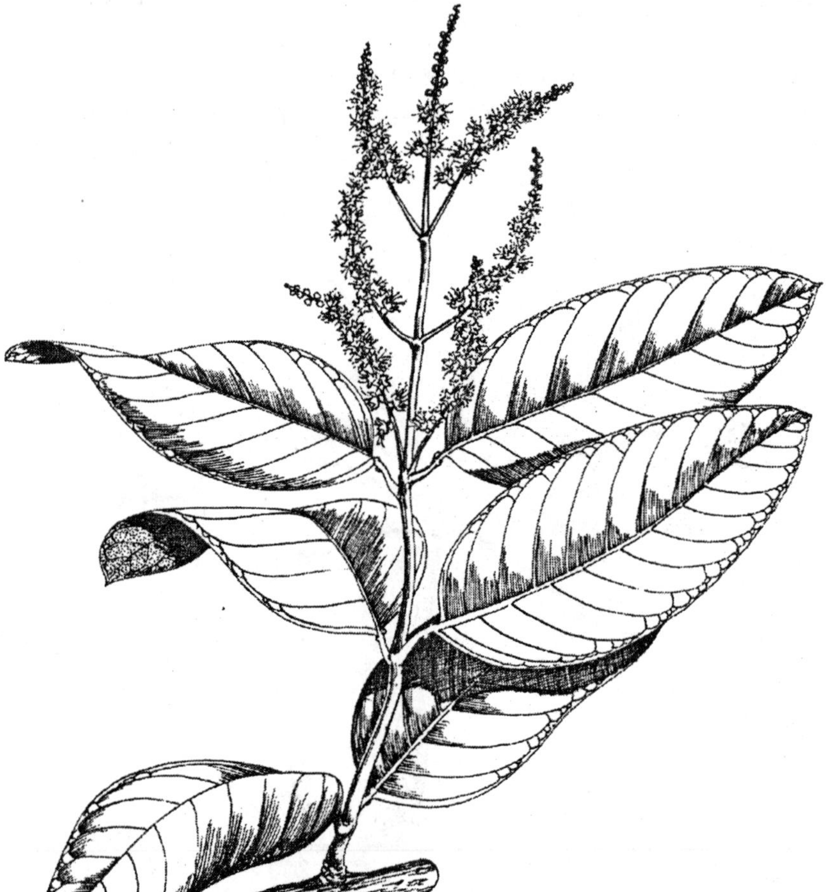

Fig. 86. *Terminalia chebula* Retz.

Themeda quadrivalvis (Linn.) O. Ktze. (Poaceae) *Godi ghass*

Tall, erect, geniculately branched perennial grass; leaves linear, acute; ligule long, membranous; panicle dense. Common along the bank of rivers, streams, at the foot of hills and in open grassy plains. Fl. & Fr.: September - November.

Small fishes with whole plant of *Themeda quadrivalvis* are fed to the animal to treat flatulence.

Tinospora cordifolia **(Willd.) Miers (Menispermaceae)** *Giloy, Neem - giloi* (Plate 8)

Succulent glabrous, deciduous climber, with corky and lenticelled bark; leaves ovate - cordate; flowers in axillary raceme; fruits globose. Common among hedges, particularly in hilly area. Fl. & Fr.: December-June.

Decoction of 50 g *Tinospora cordifolia* (whole plant) and a spoonful of powder of dried rhizome of *Curcuma longa* is given orally twice in a day upto three days to treat tonsillitis as well as foot and mouth disease. Paste of about 100 g roots is given once in a day upto five days to increases the secretion of milk. Paste of about 150 g stem is given twice in a day upto five days to the animal to treat haematuria. Extract of whole plant is given to the animal to treat general weakness. Extract of whole plant is given to bulls to increase the sexual power.

Trachyspermum ammi **(Linn.) Sprague (Apiaceae)** *Ajwain*

Annual herb; flowers whitish or pinkish; fruits muricate, sub - hispid. Widely cultivated for the fruits which are used as condiment. Fl. & Fr.: November- March.

About 80 to 100 g seeds are powdered and given with jaggery upto two days in oestrus induction.

Trianthema portulacastrum **Linn. (Aizoaceae)** *Kala - Satta*

Succulent, prostrate herb; leaves spathulate; flowers white or pink, solitary; stamens ten. Common in waste places and cultivated fields. Fl. & Fr.: September - November.

Paste of 250 g leaves of *Trianthema portulacastrum* and 10 g seeds of *Piper nigrum* (pepper) is given orally to treat diarrhoea.

Tribulus terrestris **Linn. (Zygophyllaceae)** *Gokhru, Pili- kante*

Prostrate to procumbent annual, hairy herb; leaves pinnate; flowers yellow; mericarps dorsally tuberculate; spines 4. Abundant in open wastelands in sandy and gravelly soils. Fl. & Fr.: August – December.

About 250 g shoots of this plant are given with fodder for two days for removal of internal parasites. Paste of about 25 g roots and 25 g leaves of *Azadirachta indica* (Neem) is applied locally to remove external parasites. Fruits are given to the animal with fodder to treat diarrhoea.

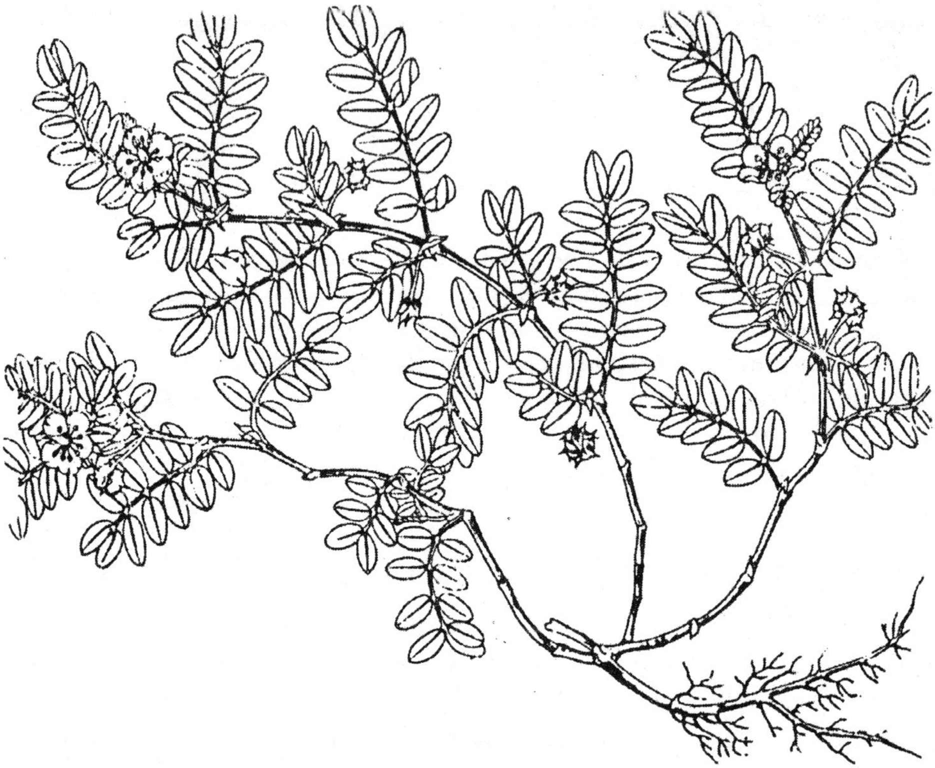

Fig. 87. *Tribulus terrestris* Linn.

***Trichodesma indica* (Linn.) R. Br. (Boraginaceae)** *Sial Kanto*

Erect or diffused herb; stem sparsely covered by trichomes; leaves distant, chartaceous, glabrous beneath, with tubercle - based trichomes above. Common in open wastelands. Fl. & Fr.: July – November.

Leaf extract is given to treat fever and bodyache.

***Trichosanthes anguina* Linn. (Cucurbitaceae)** *Charchenda*

Annual climbers. Leaves 8-14 by 10-16 cm, broadly ovate-cordate or orbicular-reniform, denticulate, 3 to 5 angled or lobed, scabrid on both the surface; tendrils 2 to 3 fid; flowers white, bracts minute, entire; fruits 25-80 cm long, often coiled, smooth with 7-8 white stripes along the length; seeds 15 by 8 mm, oblong, finely rugulose, undulate. Occasionally found in wastelands, particularly on the boundaries of fields and gardens. Fl. & Fr.: July – October.

100 g root , 100 g onion, 250 g curd and 150 g salt is given orally thrice in a day to treat gastritis.

Trichosanthes bracteata **(Lam.) Voigt (Cucurbitaceae)**
Kakighado

Extensive climber; leaves membranous, broadly ovate-cordate, 3- to 5-angled; tendril robust, sulcate; flowers white, villose-hirsute; fruit bright red; seeds peculiar, transversely broad, belted at the middle, belt with raised margins. Rare, in wastelands and open forests. Fl. & Fr.: July- October

Root extract is given to animalsthrough drenching tube to treat flatulence.

Trichosanthes cucumerina **Linn. (Cucurbitaceae)** *Indrani, Jangli- chichinda, Kechan*

Annual climber; leaves broadly ovate or orbicular-reniform, denticulate, deeply 5 to 7-lobed; tendril slender, 2- to 3-fid; flower white; fruits 8-10 seeded; seeds ovate-oblong, compressed, undulate, truncate, base attenute. Common in the east of Aravalli; particularly in wastelands. Fl. & Fr.: August-October

Decoction of 50 g roots is given orally once in a day upto two days to treat vulvo-vaginal uterine prolapse. Fruit juice is given to the animal through drenching tube to treat urinary diseases.

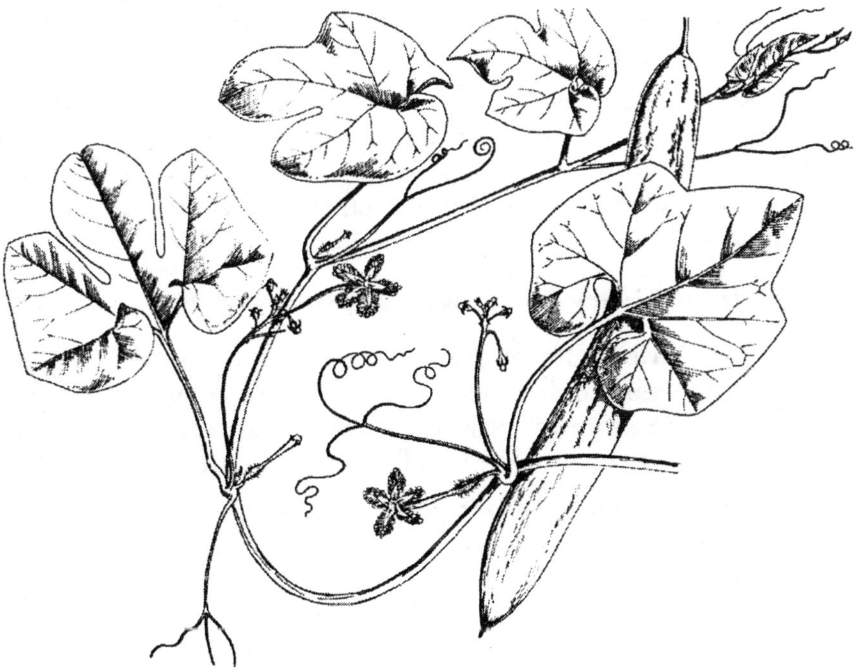

Fig. 88. *Trichosanthes cucumerina* Linn.

Tridax procumbens **Linn. (Asteraceae)** *Tokariyo, Pebula ka mocha, Kalal* (Plate 8)

Straggling herb; leaves ovate - lanceolate; heads yellow, terminating long peduncles; achenes silky. Common among bushes in wasteland. Fl. & Fr.: Most part of the year.

Infusion of 100 g dried leaves is given orally to treat diarrhoea. Fresh leaf extract or paste is applied on the wounds and cuts of animal to treat bleeding.

Trigonella foenum - graecum **Linn. (Fabaceae)** *Methi*

Herb; leaves 3 - foliolate; pale yellow flowers; pods straight, turgid beaked. Cultivated for the seeds used as condiment and leaves as vegetable. Fl. & Fr.: November- March

Infusion of 1 kg seed flour is given to the animal daily upto three days to treat haematuria. Fresh leaves and seeds mixed with fodder are fed to the animal to treat rheumatism. Seeds mixed with jaggery are fed to cows and buffaloes to enhance lactation.

Triticum aestivum **Linn. (Poaceae)** *Gehu*

Medium – sized annuals, with flat leaves; inflorescence a terminal, distichous spike; spikelets solitary, awned. Widely grown for its grains and straw. Fl. & Fr.: November- March

About 500 g sprouted seeds of *Triticum aestivum* mixed with jaggery (*Saccharum officinarum*) and seed oil of *Brassica campestris* are given to the animal upto five to ten days for oestrus induction. Paste of roasted seeds is mixed with fodder and fed to goats to treat gastric problem.

Typha angustata **Bory & Chaub. (Typhaceae)** *Era, Pota, Patera*

Erect rhizomatous herb; leaves linear, spongy, flat above and convex beneath; spike cylindrical, male flowers above, female below and upto 3 mm long gap in between. Common in marshy and aquatic habitats throughout the state. Fl. & Fr.: August- June.

Poultice of inflorescence is tied on the broken horn of animal to stop bleeding. Poultice of inflorescence is also tied on the wound for its early healing.

Urena lobata **Linn. (Malvaceae)** *Roolru*

Erect, perennial herb; leaves broadly ovate - suborbicular; flowers solitary or in clusters of 2-3, in the axils of uppermost leaves;

mericarps densely clothed with hooked hairs. Common along roads in waste places and forest edges. Fl. & Fr.: September – January.

Leaf extract is used to treat wounds. Decoction of roots is given orally to animal to treat diarrhoea.

Urginea indica **(Roxb.) Kunth (Liliaceae)** *Jangli- kanda, Koli-kanda, Jangli- piaz* (Plate 8)

Scapigerous, perennial herb; with ovoid, tunicated bulbs; leaves radical, flat, linear; flowers few, born on long scapes; capsule triquetrous. Common in gravelly and rocky habitats. Fl. & Fr.: February - May

Bulbs are fed to the animal upto seven to eight days with fodder to treat mastitis (*'Thanella'*).

Vanda tessellata **(Roxb.) Hook. ex G. Don (Orchidaceae)** *Va - Hankal, Akashvel, Hawai* (Plate 8)

Epiphytic; stem sheathed; leaves patent, recurved, coriaceous, linear - oblong, strap - shaped, unequally 2- 3 dented at the apex, flowers in racemes; capsule oblong, winged. Common epiphytic, mostly on trees in dry deciduous forest. It is also seen on semi evergreen forest. Fl. & Fr.: May- June

Decoction of whole plant is given to the animal to treat hysteria.

Vernonia cinerea **Linn. (Asteraceae)** *Kali jeeri*

Erect or decumbent, annual – perennial herbs, 5-100 cm high; stems ribbed; leaves 0.5-8.0 by 0.3-3.5 cm, variable in shape from ovate to obovate. Common in variable habitats Fl. & Fr.: Most part of the year.

Seeds are given to the animal to treat food-poisoning. Infusion of seeds is give to the animal upto three days to treat fever.

Vernonia anthelmintica **(Linn.) Willd. (Asteraceae)** *Kalijiri*

Erect, aromatic, gland punctuate or glandular hairy, annual herbs. Leaves sessile, 4-6 by 2.0-2.5 cm, elliptic-obovate or ovate. Common in wet and shaded habitats in wastelands and forests. Fl. & Fr.: January-March.

About 250 g seeds of *Trachyspermum ammi* ('Ajwain'), 250 g dried rhizomes of *Curcuma longa* (Haldi), 100 g seeds of *Vernonia anthel-*

mintica (Kalijiri) and 2 kg jaggery are mixed properly and bolus of about 150 g are prepared and fed to the animal to treat fever.

***Vigna aconitifolia* Jacq. (Fabaceae)** *Moth*

Erect or diffuse, glabrous herb; leaves 3-foliolate, leaflets palmatipartite, 3.5-6.0 cm long; flowers in axillary, yellow; seeds oblong, smooth, brown. Common in open wastelands and grassland. Fl. & Fr.: August-January.

About 250 g seed flour is mixed with salt and butter milk and fed to the animal to treat diarrhoea.

***Vitis vitiginea* Haines (Vitaceae)** *Jangli - angoor*

Weak climber; simple cordate leaves; flowers in umbellate compound cymes; fruits pale - purple. Rare, outskirts of forests and boundaries of field. Fl. & Fr.: August – November.

Extract of aerial part is given orally to animals through drenching tube in bronchitis. The root decoction is applied to treat boils.

***Vitex negundo* Linn. (Verbenaceae)** *Nagad, Nirgundi* (Plate 8)

Evergreen shrub; tender part whitish grey, pubescent; leaves 3- to 5- foliolate; flowers violet or blue in terminal, long panicles; drupes ovoid, 4- celled, each cell with one seed, enclosed by persistant calyx. Very common along the streams and riverbeds. Fl. & Fr.: Almost throughout the year.

Paste of 50 g tender leaves of *Vitex negundo* with 5 g seed powder of *Piper nigrum* and four to five bulbs of *Allium sativum* is given to treat ephemeral fever and impaction. Paste of leaves is applied locally as an ointment to treat skin disease. It is also applied on the eyes to treat conjunctivitis.

***Withania somnifera* (Linn.) Dunal (Solanaceae)** *Padalsi, Ashgandh.*

Much branched under shrub, clothed with greenish - white hairs; leaves ovate or ovate - oblong; flowers clustered in axillary, subsessile, umbellate cymes; berries globose, orange - red, enclosed in 5 - angled, pubescent, apiculate, membranous cover of inflated calyx. Common in dry wastelands, preferably in fertile soil. Fl. & Fr.: Most part of the year.

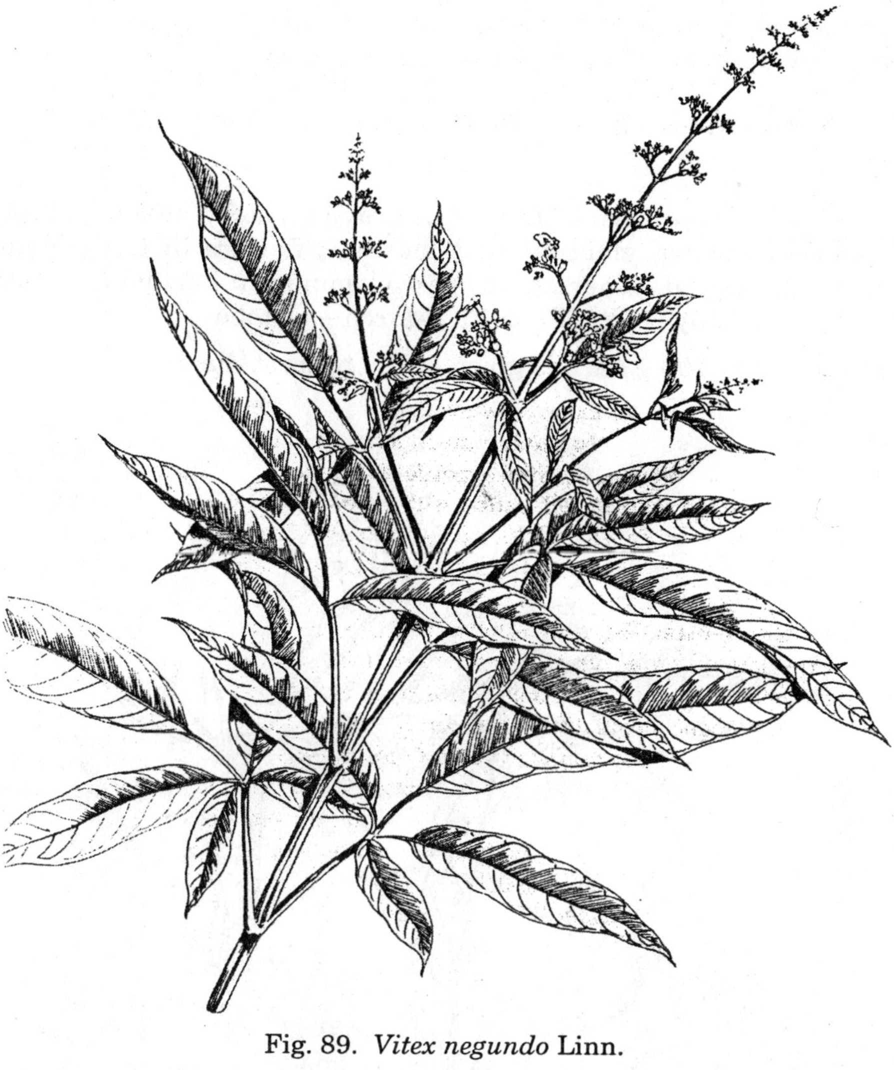

Fig. 89. *Vitex negundo* Linn.

Paste of root or stem of *Withania somnifera* is applied on the skinto treat bacterial infection. Decoction of 1 kg roots and 2 litres sesamum oil is given to the animals to treat lumbago.

***Woodfordia fruticosa* (Linn.) Kuntz (Lythraceae)** *Ban-mahendi, Dhavdi* (Plate 8)

Straggling deciduous shrub; leaves sessile, broadly lanceolate, hoary-tomentose, nigro-punctate beneath; flowers axillary or extra axillary, in fascicled cymes; capsule oblong, shining brown; seeds minute, narrowly obconical-trigonous cuneate at base. Common in the forests, on the walls of old buildings and in wastelands. Fl. & Fr.: January – June.

Decoction of flowers is used to treat wound. 50 g root extract is given orally upto 10 -15 days to treat rheumatism.

Wrightia tinctoria **(Roxb.) R. Br. (Apocynaceae)** *Kheer, Khani, Khirni*

Deciduous tree; bark fissured, grayish-black; leaves elliptic-lanceolate or oblong, glabrous or pubescent; flowers in trichotomous cymes; fruits paired, cohering at apex. Common in deciduous forests, particularly in hilly tracts. Fl. & Fr.: March – October.

Decoction of 100 g bark is given orally to treat diarrhoea.

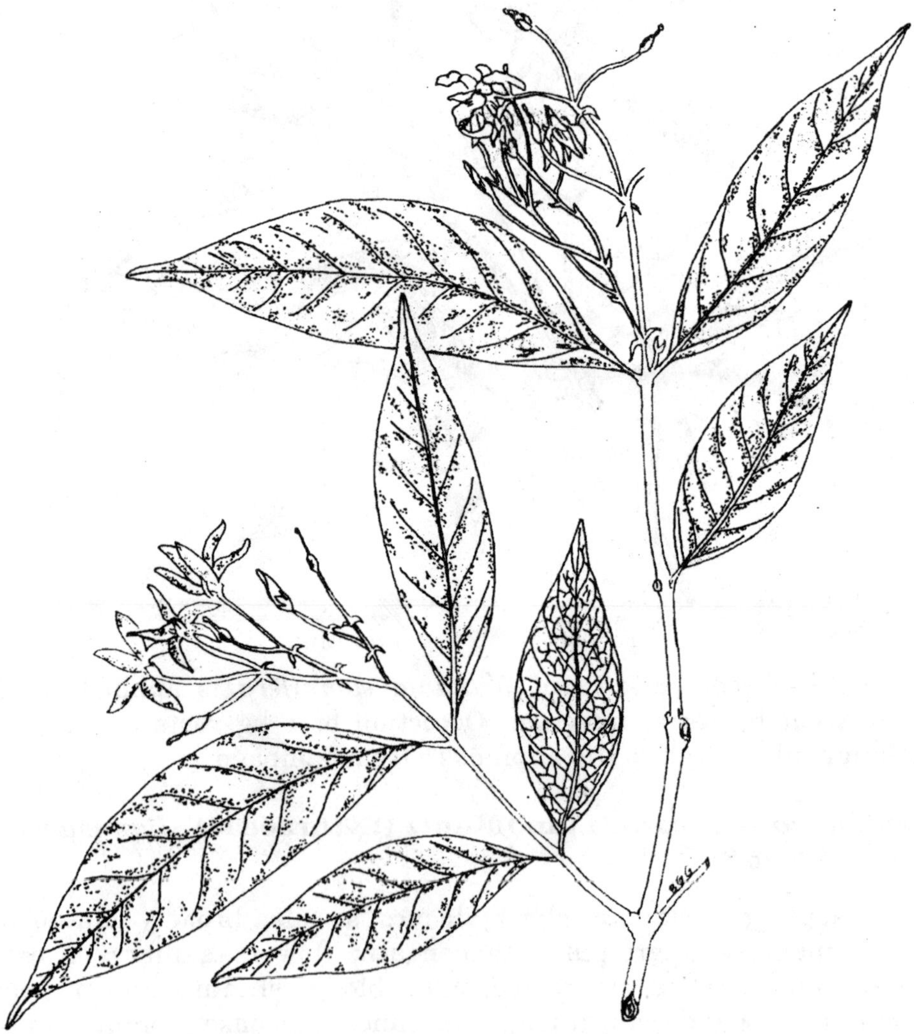

Fig. 90. *Wrightia tinctoria* (Roxb.) R. Br.

***Xanthium strumarium* Linn. (Asteraceae)** *Jhadugar, Bichhu-butti*

Erect, annual, upto 120 cm high, foetid - smelling unarmed herb; leaves ovate - suborbicular; head in terminal and axillary racemes. Found very commonly in waste places, near ditches, ponds etc. Fl. & Fr.: October –December.

Paste of leaf is applied on the wound to kill the maggots.

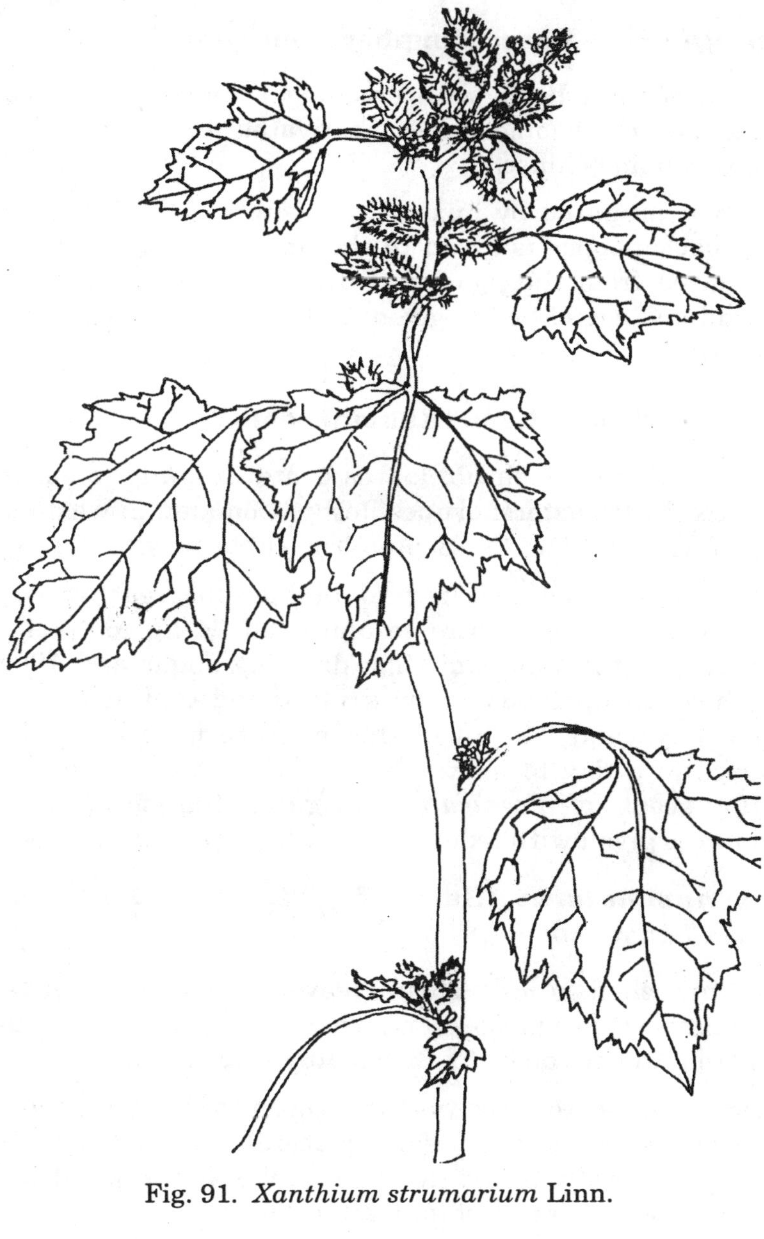

Fig. 91. *Xanthium strumarium* Linn.

***Zea mays* Linn. (Poaceae)** *Makki, Makka*

Monoecious annual; male spikelets usually in terminal racemes; female inflorescence consists of many spikelets seated on a spongy axis. Cultivated during rainy season for its grains. Fl. & Fr.: November - February

Decoction of 100 g roots is given orally upto five/seven days to cure weakness after delivery.

***Zingiber officinale* Rosc. (Zingiberaceae)** *Adrak, Ada*

Erect, perennial herb; with creeping tuberous rhizomes; leaves subsessile; flowers in long spikes. Cultivated for its edible rhizomes. Fl. & Fr.: November- March.

Decoction prepared by mixing 250 g milk fat, 10 g dried ginger and 10 g black pepper is given to the animal to treat stomachache. Bolus prepared from the powder of dried *Zingiber officinale, Allium sativum* and one egg of hen is given to the animal to treat pneumonia and paralysis.

***Ziziphus mauritiana* Lam. (Rhamnaceae)** *Bor*

Erect small tree or shrub; leaves ovate - elliptic to suborbicular; flowers in axillary clusters; drupes fleshy. Common in wastelands and ourstrike of forests. Fl. & Fr.: September – February.

Seeds are grinded and fed to buffalo to treat vulvo-vaginal-uterine prolapse. About 2 litre sesamum-oil, ½ kg roots of *Ziziphus mauritiana*, 100 g Ammonium chloride, 2 kg sugar and 100g clay is mixed with wheat husk and water is added and kept in an earthen pot upto three days and 750 ml of this mixture is given orally to the animal once in a day to induce lactation.Mixture of 50g *'lac'* of this plant, 10g seeds of *Foeniculum vulgare*, 10g seeds of *Ocimum americanum* is given with fodder to treat leucorrhoea and heat-stroke.

***Ziziphus nummularia* (Burm. f.) Wt. & Arn. (Rhamnaceae)** *Jhar - bor, Chania - bor*

Much branched, prickly shrub; leaves orbicular-ovate; flowers in axillary cymes; drupes globose, red when ripe. Common in wastelands especially in desertic zones. Fl. & Fr.: July – January.

Decoction of two to three years old thorns of *Ziziphus nummularia* is given to the animal for disposal of placenta after delivery. Decoction of roots is given orally to induce labour pain. Whole plant is fed with fodder to increase secretion of milk after delivery.

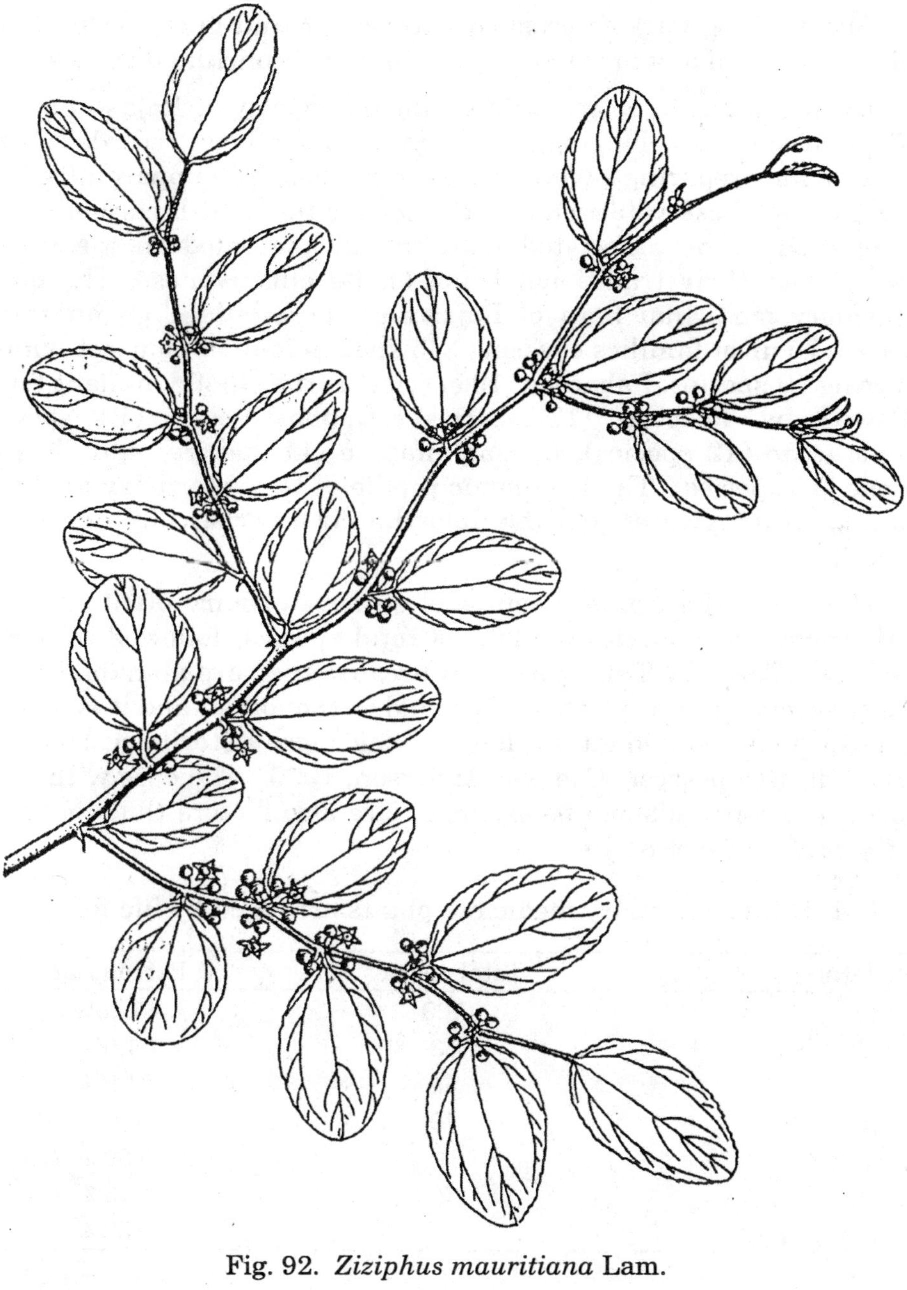

Fig. 92. *Ziziphus mauritiana* Lam.

***Ziziphus xylopyra* (Retz.) Willd. (Rhamnaceae)** *Gatori, Ghat bor*

Erect tree or straggling shrub; leaves elliptic oblong, stipular prickles paired; flower greenish, covered with dense, grey tomentum. Occasionally found in mixed deciduous forests at low altitude and in wastelands.

About 250 g bark is crushed with water and given orally to the animal once in a day four to five days to treat bronchial diseases.

During the exhaustive ethnomedicinal survey of Rajasthan, total 265 plant species belonging to 91 families have been recorded, which are used for preparing several herbal remedies. The apparent reliance of tribals on these veterinary medicines for the health care of animal is reported to be associated with the lack of modern medication, poverty and their traditional belief on its effectiveness. The ethnoveterinary medicinal flora of Rajasthan represents 1 Gymnosp-erm species, 75 dicot families covering 215 species and 16 monocot families covering 49 species. Fabaceae (19 species) is the chief dominant family followed by Poaceae (17 species), Euphorbiaceae (12 species), Mimosaceae (12 species), Caesalpiniaceae (11 species) and Cucurbitaceae (11 species). The taxonomic profile of the veterinary medicinal plant species indicates that the Rajasthan is a floristically rich area of India.

Herbs are the primary source of ethnoveterinary plants in terms of the number of species (45.28% of total species) followed by shrubs and trees (Table 1). This is perhaps because they are abundant and/or weedy species that are frequently found in the forest, and it is believed that the more abundant a plant is, the more veterinary medicinal virtues it may possess (Coe and Anderson, 1996). The ease with which bioactive compounds can be extracted are also factors that contribute to the preference of herbs.

Table 1. Ethnoveterinary medicinal plants arranged by life form

Life form	Total species	Percentage
Herbs	120	45.28%
Shrubs	63	31.5%
Trees	58	21.8%
Climbers	19	7.1%
Epiphyte	1	0.39%
Parasite	3	1.13%
Gymnosperm	1	0.39%

Plant parts used

The plant parts used for the veterinary drug preparations are bark, flowers, fruits, leaves, rhizomes, roots, sap, seeds, stems and young shoots. In some cases the whole plant including the roots are utilized.

Ailments treated

Gastro-intestinal problems, maternity ailments, skin diseases, skelto - muscular problems, animal bites, internal and external parasites etc. are the most frequent ailments treated with the ethnoveterinary medicial plants. Most of the species are found having more than a single therapeutic use. The largest number of plants (91 plants) are used to treat gastro-intestinal ailments (constipation, diarrhoea/dysentery, gastric, flatulence, indigestion, stomachache), 69 are used for maternity ailments, 54 plants are used to treat skin diseases, 42 plants are used to treat skeleto - muscular problems and 29 plants are used to treat animal bites, internal and external parasites. Diseases like foot and mouth disease, horn breakage, ENT, sun stroke etc. are also common and to a lesser extent for ophthalmological ailments, fever, cardiovascular diseases and genito urinary ailments etc. (Table 2 and 3).

Table 2. Major disease categories and botanical name of ethnoveterinary medicinal plants used to treat various ailments

Disease category	Name of Plants used to treat veterinary diseases
Animal bites, internal and external parasites	: *Adhatoda zeylanica, Aerva lanata, Alternanthera pungens,*
	: *Alangium salvifolium, Annona squamosa, Apluda mutica, Balanites aegyptiaca, Butea monosperma, Blumea lacera, Calotropis procera, Cardiospermum halicacabum, Cissampelos pareira, Cleome viscosa, Clerodendrum phlomidis, Cocculus hirsutus, Curculigo orchioides, Dendrocalamus strictus, Elytraria acaulis, Fagonia indica, Ferula asafoetida, Imperata cylindrica, Melia azedarach, Momordica dioica, Sarcostemma viminale, Sesbania aculeata, Shorea robusta, Tephrosia purpurea, Tribulus terrestris* and *Xanthium strumarium.*
Skeleto – muscular problems (Bone fracture)	: *Acacia leucophloea, Acacia pennata, Aegle marmelos, Aerva pseudotomentosa, Allium sativum, Ampelocissus latifolia, Aristolochia bracteolata, Bauhinia purpurea, Bombax ceiba, Boswellia serrata, Butea monosperma, Calotropis gigantea, Capparis decidua, Capparis sepiaria, Carissa congesta, Cassia auriculata, Cissus quadrangularis, Cleome viscosa, Clerodendrum phlomidis, Commelina forsskalaei, Commiphora wightii, Costus speciosus, Curculigo orchioides, Curcuma longa, Curcuma aromatica, Cuscuta reflexa, Dendrocalamus strictus, Ficus benghalensis, Grewia damine, Grewia tenax, Guizotia oleifera, Jatropha curcas, Jatropha gossypifolia, Leea macrophylla, Martynia annua, Pithecellobium dulce, Sarcostemma viminale, Sida ovata, Trigonella foenum – graecum, Withania*

somnifera, Woodfordia fruticosa and *Zingiber officinale.*

Fever : *Adhatoda zeylanica, Allium sativum, Anogeissus latifolia, Aristolochia bracteolata, Caesalpinia bonduc, Citrullus colocynthis, Cleome viscosa, Curcuma amada, Cymbopogon martini, Enicostema axillare, Euphorbia fusiformis, Grewia orientalis, Leucas aspera, Phyllanthus fraternus, Phyllanthus virgatus, Piper betel, Portulaca oleracea, Shorea robusta, Trichodesma indica, Vernonia cinerea, Vernonia anthelmintica, Vitex negundo* and *Ziziphus mauritiana.*

ENT : *Adhatoda zeylanica, Argyreia nervosa, Capparis sepiaria, Capsicum annum, Coccinia grandis, Corallocarpus epigaeus, Datura metel, Manilkara hexandra, Mimosa pudica* and *Tinospora cordifolia.*

Opthalmological ailments : *Achyranthes aspera, Albizia lebbeck, Coccinia grandis, Jatropha curcas, Soymida febrifuga* and *Vitex negundo.*

Gastro – intestinal ailments : *Abrus precatorius, Abutilon indicum, Achyranthes aspera, Adhatoda zeylanica, Aegle marmelos, Aerva lanata, Aerva pseudotomentosa, Ailanthus excelsa, Anisomeles indica, Annona squamosa, Arisaema tortuosum, Arundo donax, Bauhinia racemosa, Boswellia serrata, Brassica campestris, Brassica juncea, Butea monosperma, Caesalpinia bonduc, Calligonum polygonoides, Capsicum minimum, Cassia angustifolia, Cassia auriculata, Cassia fistula, Catunaregam spinosa, Chlorophytum tuberosum, Cicer arietinum, Citrullus colocynthis, Cleome viscosa, Clitoria ternatea, Corchorus depressus, Cordia dichotoma, Coriandrum sativum, Cosmostigma racemosa, Crotalaria burhia, Cucumis callosus, Curcuma amada, Cyamopsis tatragonoloba, Dalbergia sissoo, Delonix elata, Desmostachya bipinnata, Digitaria adscendens, Diospyros melanoxylon, Echinops echinatus, Elytraria acaulis, Ephedra ciliata, Euphorbia fusiformis, Euphorbia hirta, Euphorbia neriifolia, Ferula asafetida, Helicteres isora, Heteropogon contortus, Jatropha curcas, Jatropha gossypifolia, Leea macrophylla, Leptadenia pyrotechnica, Luffa acutangula, Luffa echinata, Mangifera indica, Nicotiana tabacum, Nyctanthes arbor – tristis, Nymphaea nauchali, Ougeinia oogeinsis, Parkinsonia aculeata, Pedalium murex, Pennisetum typhoidis, Piper betel, Plumbago zeylanica, Prosopis cineraria, Pterocarpus marsupium, Pupalia atropurpurea, Ricinus communis, Salvia aegyptiaca, Sesamum indicum, Shorea robusta, Sorghum halepense, Soymida febrifuga, Syzygium cumini, Tamarindus indica, Tephrosia purpurea, Terminalia bellirica, Terminalia chebula, Themeda quadrivalvis, Trianthema portulacastrum, Trichosanthes anguina, Trichosanthes bracteata, Tridax procumbens, Triticum aestivum, Urena lobata, Vigna aconitifolia, Wrightia tinctoria* and *Zingiber officinale.*

Genito-urinary ailment : *Abutilon indicum, Aerva javanica, Bombax ceiba, Calligonum polygonoides, Ceropegia attenuata, Cuscuta reflexa, Dalbergia sissoo, Ficus religiosa, Hibiscus rosa- sinensis, Tinospora cordifolia, Trichosanthes cucumerina* and *Trigonella foenum – graecum.*

Liver disorder : *Alangium salvifolium*

Maternity ailments : *Abrus precatorius, Acacia catechu, Acacia leucophloea, Acacia nilotica, Achyranthes aspera, Aeschynomene aspera, Amaranthus spinosus, Anethum graveolens, Anisomeles indica, Asparagus racemosus, Azadirachta indica, Bidens biternata, Blepharis linariaefolia, Bombax ceiba, Butea monosperma, Caesalpinia bonduc, Cassia tora, Chlorophytum tuberosum, Citrullus colocynthis, Citrus medica, Cocculus pendulus, Corchorus depressus, Cordia dichotoma, Crotalaria burhia, Cucumis callosus, Curcuma amada, Curcuma longa, Datura innoxia, Dendrophthoe falcata, Dichrostachys cinerea, Dioscorea bulbifera, Echinops echinatus, Elettaria cardamomum, Eleusine coracana, Enicostema axillare, Euphorbia caducifolia, Euphorbia heyneana, Euphorbia neriifolia, Ferula asafoetida, Ficus religiosa, Gossypium herbaceum, Gloriosa superba, Hibiscus rosa- sinensis, Jatropha gossypifolia, Lagenaria siceraria, Leptadenia pyrotechnica, Leptadenia reticulata, Lycium barbarum, Madhuca indica, Mentha spicata, Mucuna pruriens, Musa paradisiaca, Ocimum americanum, Pandanus fascicularis, Panicum miliaceum, Pergularia daemia, Phoenix sylvestris, Peperomia pellucida, Polygonum plebeium, Saccharum officinarum, Solanum virginianum, Sorghum vulgare, Tinospora cordifolia, Trachyspermum ammi, Trichosanthes cucumerina, Triticum aestivum, Urginea indica, Ziziphus mauritiana* and *Ziziphus nummularia.*

Paralysis and Hysteria : *Bacopa monnieri Celastrus paniculata* and *Vanda tessellata.*

Respiratory tract infection : *Adhatoda zeylanica, Ailanthus excelsa, Fagonia indica, Jatropha curcas, Lycium barbarum, Ocimum americanum, Vitis vitiginea, Zingiber officinale* and *Ziziphus xylopyra.*

Skin diseases and related Ailments : *Adhatoda zeylanica, Ageratum conyzoides, Aloe vera, Anardium occidentale, Argemone mexicana, Argyreia nervosa, Barleria prionitis, Bauhinia racemosa, Biophytum sensitivum, Brassica campestris, Caesalpinia bonduc, Calotropis procera, Carica papaya, Cassia auriculata, Ceropegia bulbosa, Chenopodium album, Cleome gynandra, Coccinia grandis, Crinum asiaticum, Curcuma aromatica, Dalbergia sissoo, Dioscorea alata, Euphorbia fusiformis, Euphorbia trucalli, Ficus carica, Ficus racemosa, Gardenia turgida, Hemidesmus indicus, Holarrhena pubescens, Holoptelea integrifolia, Indigofera linifolia,*

	Kalanchoe pinnata, Lawsonia inermis, Lindernia crustacean, Mirabilis jalapa, Moringa oleifera, Nerium oleander, Ocimum tenuiflorum, Polygonum plebeium, Pongamia pinnata, Prosopis juliflora, Rhus mysurensis, Saccharum officinarum, Salvadora oleoides, Sesamum indicum, Solanum virginianum, Tecomella undulata, Tectona grandis, Tridax procumbens, Typha angustata, Urena lobata, Vitis vitiginea, Vitex negundo and *Woodfordia fruticosa.*
Foot and mouth disease	: *Acacia nilotica, Aerva pseudotomentosa, Allium sativum, Anisomeles indica, Annona squamosa, Bauhinia variegate, Butea monosperma, Cissus quandrangula, Cordia dichotoma, Curculigo orchioides, Gloriosa superba, Hygrophila auriculata, Pergularia daemia, Phaseolus mungo, Sesamum indicum,* and *Tinospora cordifolia.*
Horn breakage	: *Aerva javanica, Agave Americana, Asparagus racemosus, Brassica campestris* and *Mallotus philippensis.*
Food poisoning	: *Acacia concinna, Celosia argentea, Curcuma aromatica, Leea macrophylla* and *Vernonia cinerea.*
General weakness	: *Acacia nilotica, Allium cepa, Allium sativum, Crotalaria juncea, Leucas cephalotes, Mimosa hamata, Pandanus fascicularis, Sorghum halepense, Terminallia arjuna, Tinospora cordifolia* and *Zea mays.*
Deficiency diseases	: *Allium cepa* and *Pueraria tuberosa.*
Bovine viral mammaitis (BVM)	: *Cistanche tubulosa.*
Infection in hooves	: *Garuga pinnata* and *Ougeinia oojeinensis.*
Anthrax	: *Holarrhena pubescens*
Carries in teeth	: *Sida ovata*

Table 3. Major disease categories and number of ethnoveterinary medicinal plants used to treat various ailments.

S.No.	Disease category	No. of plants used to treat diseases
1	Animal bites, internal and external parasites	29
2	Anthrax	1
3	Bovine viral mammaitis (BVM)	1
4	Carries in teeth	1
5	General weakness	10
6	Deficiency diseases	2
7	ENT	10
8	Fever	23
9	Food poisoning	5
10	Foot and mouth disease	16
11	Gastro – intestinal ailments	91

12	Genito-urinary ailment	13
13	Horn breakage	5
14	Infection in hooves	2
15	Liver disorders	1
16	Maternity ailments	69
17	Ophthalmological ailments	6
18	Paralysis and Hysteria	3
19	Respiratory tract infection	9
20	Sexual weakness	1
21	Skeleto – muscular problems (Bone fracture)	42
22	Skin diseases and related ailments	54

Knowledge of plants and treatment

Most of the people interviewed were familiar with the species dealing with common ailments like digestive problems, fever, and skin diseases. In tribal communities, common knowledge about ethnoveterinary herbs was learned from the elders and community members who share knowledge about mode of collection and administration of ethnoveterinary medicinal plants. However, the knowledge of ethnoveterinary plants for complex problems associated with maternity problems and urinary infection were confined only to a few families or people, some of which serve as local healers and veterinary medicine men. This kind of curative information was kept with some sanctity and secrecy, with the belief that the medicines would lose their potency if revealed to other people.

Administration of medicines

Medical administration included oral absorption, poultice and paste applying, rubbing and massage. Most of the ailments such as gastro-intestinal disorder and maternity ailment can be treated by oral absorption while most of the skin diseases can be treated by the external application. Some ailments may be treated by both external as well as internal application such as animal bites and skeleto-muscular problems.

All other preparations mentioned here are very effective and cheaply available in the area and are used by the tribals as alternative to allopathic medicines. The treatments however show no side effects. Further research on scientific line will help in developing effective and cheap drugs for animal health care. Experimental work followed by field test can be expected to yield useful data and some additional recipes for animal health.

Tribals, for their survival in the ecosystem, based on their generations of practical experience, have evolved means and options in the form of indigenous animal health care practices that have minimal dependence on external input. These practices have helped in conservation of above-mentioned plants and sustain people themselves in the inhospitable and resource scarce ecosystem.

The indigenous animal health care practices mitigate the inadequacy in modern veterinary infrastructure, ensure resource conservation and save expenditure through minimal or least investment. Therefore, it is imperative to maintain bio-resources so that these practices are also continued.

Tribals residing in the remote forest areas of Rajasthan have an amazingly good understanding of the uses of medicinal plant parts and quantities needed, and the methods used in harvesting, processing, storing, preserving and utilizing medicinal plants to ensure good drug efficacy and to enhance the survival of plant germplasm. If the above procedures are poorly executed, plant resources may be over-exploited, which can lead to extinction of certain species. This means that the best results from medicinal plant preparations can only be obtained when the tribals and rural people are taught to judiciously harvest, process, store, preserve and utilize the preparations.

The ethnoveterinary medicinal plants listed here are locally available and easily accessible and thus provide a cheaper treatment as compared to western drugs. The only limitation is the seasonal availability of certain plants, for which tribals have acquired different ways to preserve them for off-season uses. Most common way of preserving is sun-drying.

Tribals use these medicines against various ailments to treat their suffering animals. There is no specific treatment for a particular type of animal e.g. cattle, goats, sheep, camels or horses. Same treatment is applied to different animals but the dose depends on body weight of the animal. Wherever there is a medicine specific to a particular animal, it has been specially mentioned. For example, in case of goats, leaves of *Ceropegia bulbosa* are given as fodder as a prophylactic measure against tumour formation.

Generally, it was observed that there is a certain overlap between plants used for human and animal medicine. Certain plants like *Albizia lebbeck* (conjunctivitis), *Helicteres isora* (diarrhoea), *Alangium salvifolium* (malarial fever), *Anethum graveolens* (as galactogogue), *Enicostema axillare* (fever), *Euphorbia triculii* (skin disorders), *Ricinus communis* (constipation), *Tridax procumbens* (as a blood coagulant) are used as medicine for same diseases in human beings as well as animals although the dose in such cases varies greatly. This may be possible as a result of tribal's tendency to try human medicines on animals or viz. such medicines are found to be equally useful in veterinary diseases.

Ethnoveterinary medicines can provide an opportunity of new drug research for human use also. For example, Rwandan cattle raisers used a preparation made from *Neorautanenia mitis* to treat mange, a disease caused by mites that burrow under the animal's skin. Scientists found that this plant contained an ingredient that kills the mites. They were able to make an ointment for human beings as an alternative providing low cost alternative to imported drugs. Therefore, the plants reported here may be clinically tested for their possible use in human medicine also.

It is interesting to note that certain plants/ plant parts in small quantities are useful as ethnoveterinary medicines whereas in large quantities they are poisonous and are fatal *e.g.*, *Abrus precatorius, Melia azedarach, Jatropa gossypifolia, Gloriosa superba, Butea monosperma* etc. Correct understanding of dosage of such plants may be useful in identifying their utility in ethnoveterinary medicine.

From the present study it was concluded that for acute, life threatening infections and epidemics, modern medicine such as antibiotics will remain the first choice. But for common and chronic conditions like skin diseases, worms, wounds, diarrhoea etc. ethnoveterinary medicines can be an alternative or complement to modern treatments especially because some antibiotics and other drugs have been overused, stimulating resistance among micro-organisms and leaving dangerous residues in meat, milk and groundwater. A combination of modern and local remedies and management practices might be the best for problems like ticks and trypanosomiasis where neither modern nor ethnoveterinary medicine alone provides a satisfactory solution.

To date, the communities are directing forest use to meet the needs of fodder, fuelwood, and timber through their management prescription in the operational plan for the community forestry. However, these forests also have commercially exploitable medicinal species, which are used to treat diseases both in human beings and animals. If these species are managed properly, they can serve a sustainable income source for these communities. Constraints to include medicinal plants in the operational plans are related to: the peculiarity of such resources and their distribution across a range of land uses; their seasonal availability; the difficulty of establishing sustainable harvesting methods; inadequate knowledge of techniques for proper population assessments and the lack of financial resources. However, without management prescriptions, illegal and over exploitation of commercially exploited species like *Commiphora wightii, Chlorophytum borivillianum, Abrus precatorius, Bombax ceiba, Eulophia ochreata, Pueraria tuberosa, Butea monosperma, Hemidesmus indicus, Ampelocissus latifolia, Adhatoda zeylanica, Annona squamosa, Withania somnifera, Gloriosa superba, Jatropha curcas, Plumbago zeylanica, Asparagus racemosus, Buchanania lanzan, Chlorophytum tuberosum, Clerodendrum phlomidis, Momordica dioica, Leea macrophylla, Centella asiatica, Ceropegia bulbosa, Ceropegia candelabrum, Costus speciosus, Leptadenia reticulata, Ocimum canum, Oroxylum indicum, Sterculia urens, Piper longum, Plumbago zeylanica, Tecomella undulata, Dicoma tomentosa, Gisekia pharnaceoides, Tecomella undulata,* and *Terminalia chebula* have been reported. Local people in state expressed that such practices had caused decline in the abundance of these species during the last few years. However, with increasing awareness of the economic value of medicinal plants, the need to assess these resources and to incorporate their assessment in operational plans is being realized by the local user groups in the state.

The present study indicates that Rajasthan harbours a vast diversity of medicinal plants. Despite gradual socio-culture transformation, local communities still possess substantial knowledge of plants and their uses. The reliance on folk medicines for health care is associated with the lack of modern medicines and medication, poverty and traditional belief of its effectiveness. Since there is a complete lack of phyto therapeutic evidence for many of species, we recommend that phytochemical and pharmacological studies need to be carried out in order to confirm the validity of properties attributed to these species. This is particularly relevant for species with market potential beyond the state of Rajasthan. With setting up management plans for their extraction, these medicinal resources can provide for both subsistence needs and income. This, however, requires detail assessment of resource quantities, productivity potential, sustainable harvesting methods, domestication possibilities and market value of potentially promising species and importantly, equitable benefit sharing regimes. The knowledge of the use of species reported here belongs to tribal and rural people of the state. Any benefits derived from the use of this knowledge must be shared with the inhabitants of the state.

CHAPTER - 5

ETHNOVETERINARY REMEDIES: ANIMAL AND ANIMAL PRODUCTS

Since time immemorial extensive use of plants, animals and minerals has been made in traditional medicine. A lot of efforts have gone into documentation, use, identification and validation of plant based traditional medicines but studies on most of the animal based medicine are sporadic, despite the fact that traditionally many animal based drugs are administered all over the world (Pushpangdan, 1990; Neto, 1999). In Unani and Ayurvedic system of medicine there are descriptions of many animal based medications (Shukla, 1950; Ali & Mahdihassan, 1961; Wahid & Siddiqui, 1961; Puri, 1970; Vohora & Khan, 1979). It has been documented that in Unani system of medicines about 200 drugs of animal origin are described which are claimed to be beneficial for the treatment of various ailments (Sharma, 1996). Similarly in Ayurveda also there is description of use of several animal based drugs particularly from cow, buffalo, elephant, camel, ass, goat and sheep (Pandey, 1996). Entire organism or their flesh, fat, excretions, bones, teeth, feathers, hair, horns and shells are used as medicine and for other purposes. These are used either singly or in compound formulations and prepared in a variety of forms i.e. powder, ash, soups, syrup, ointments, liniments, etc.

During the ethnoveterinary survey of the study area, about 29 animal species have been documented which are used in the preparation of ethnoveterinary remedies. In the following account, animals are arranged alphabetically by zoological names followed by their English name in paranthesis, local name in itallics & mode of administration.

ENUMERATION OF ANIMAL/ ANIMAL PRODUCT BASED REMEDIES

***Acrida exaltata* (Locust)** *Tiddi*

Two to three grasshoppers along with chapatti (bread) or fodder are fed to the animal for oestrus induction. The animal will be in heat within 15 days.

Bos bubalus **(Buffalo)** *Bhains*

Skull of a dead buffalo is boiled in water and the water is given to the camel to treat flatulence and lumbago.

Bos indicus **(Cow)** *Gay*

The dried dung is burnt and ash is applied externally to treat urticaria. Butter milk is given orally as well as applied locally to treat eczema and scabies. Milk fat of cow milk is applied externally on teats to treat mastitis.

Camelus dromedaries **(Camel)** *Oont*

Skull of dead camel is burnt to ash. About 100 g of this ash is mixed with 400 g oil of *Papaver somniferum* and given orally to cow through drenching tube once in a day upto six days to treat lumbago. Skull of a dead camel is boiled in water and the water is given to the buffalo to treat flatulence and lumbago. The dried dung is burnt and ash is applied externally on stomach to treat constipation. Blood is applied externally to treat arthritis. Old bones of dead camel are burnt and ash is mixed with water and given to the animal for treating rheumatoid arthritis.

Capra capra **(Goat)** *Bakari*

Paste prepared by mixing excreta of goat with the leaves of *Cassia auriculata* is applied to treat wound.

Capra indicus **(Goat)** *Bakra*

Blood of *Capra indicus* is massaged externally to treat fractured bone.

Canis aureus **(Jackal)** *Shiyad*

Blood is massaged externally for treating arthritis of goats.

Canis familiaris **(Dog)** *Kutro*

Excreta is applied externally to treat wounds.

Cervus unicolor **(Sambhar)** *Sabar/Harnu*

Powder of antler is applied on eyes to treat eye ailments.

Columbo livia **(Pigeon)** *Kabutar*

Paste is prepared by mixing a 12 cm root piece of *Pandanus odoratissimus*, 1 kg dried excreta of pigeon, seeds of *Sesamum indicum* and 500 g jaggery. About 500 g of this paste is given once in a day for 5 days for oestrus induction. Bolus prepared from dried excreta of pigeon with jaggery is fed to the animal once in a day for oestrus induction. The blood is massaged externally to treat paralysis.

***Coracias benghalensis* (Indian roller/Blue jay)** *Neelkanth*

Four to five feathers along with fresh *Cynodon dactylon* are fed to animal for disposal of placenta after delivery.

***Corvus splendens* (Crow)** *Kagla*

One crow is hunted, boiled and fed to the animal to treat flatulence. Roasted or boiled flesh is given to treat whooping cough

***Cyanopterus sphinx* (Bat)** *'Chamachidiu'*

Raw flesh having blood is rubbed to treat external injuries and also fed to the animal to treat whooping cough.

***Equus hemionuskhur* (Indian wildass)** *Ghudkhar*

Blood of *Equus hemionuskhur* is massaged externally to treat arthritis.

***Gallus domesticus* (Hen)** *Murgi*

Shell of four to five eggs of hen are fed to buffalo once in a day up to one week for oestrus induction. Blood is externally massaged on the aching parts of body. Blood is applied externally for treating arthritis and fractured bone. Eggs of hen are given orally to animal upto 8 days for the treatment of fractured bone.

***Hemidactylus flaviviridis* (Lizard)** *Chhipkali*

One lizard is hunted and fed to the animal to treat lumbago.

***Hystrix indica* (Porcupine)** *Sehi*

About 5 g ash of hairs is given orally to treat asthma. Smoke of burning hairs is given to the animal to treat foot and mouth disease. Spines of hedgehog are collected and animals are exposed to the smoke of these spines to treat foot and mouth disease.

***Microtermes obesiholmgren* (White ant, termite)** *Dimak*

Soil of termite mounds is rubbed thoroughly up to five to ten minutes on the jaw of the animal and repeated frequently upto three days to treat poisoning caused due to feeding of immature Sorghum to the animal.

Hippocampus cuda **(Sea horse, Hippopotamus)** *Ghoda machchhi*

Dried animal is powdered and fed to the animal with fodder to treat stomachache of horses.

Hyaena hyaena **(Hyena)** *Zarakh*

Fat is applied externally to treat arthritis; blood is applied on cloth and smoke of this burning cloth is used to treat asthma.

Lepus nigricollis ruficodatum **(Rufous-tailed hare)** *Sasla*

Blood is applied externally to treat swelling; the ash of tail is mixed with oil and is applied to treat burning sensation.

Lissemys punctatus **(Indian flap, Shell turtle, Tortoise)** *Kachbo*

Carapace is burnt and ash is used for healing of internal injuries, pruritus and cough; and for treating superficial blunt injuries of animal.

***Palamneaus* sp. (Scorpion)** *Bichchhoo*

A black scorpion is caught and dipped in a bottle full of mustard oil. After some time this oil is applied locally to treat scorpion bite.

Paraechinus microlapus **(Shero)** *Palehedge hog*

Smoke of burning skin is used to treat mouth diseases of animal.

Passer domesticus **(House sparrow)** *Charkali*

Ash of excreta is used to treat asthma in calves.

Pavo cristatus **(Peafowl)** *Mor*

Legs of peafowl are boiled in oil, and used to treat the earache.

Pseudibis papillosa **(Black ibis Blood)** *Ran Kagdo*

Blood is massaged for treating burning sensation, nervous disorder, paralysis and inherent body heat.

Vespa orientalis **(Wasp)** *Tatia*

Some *Vespa orientalis* are caught and boiled with water. Steam treatment this water is given to the mammary glands of animal to treat mastitis. Paste of soil of hive is applied locally to treat swelling and mastitis.

***Quis aries* (Sheep)** *Bhed*

Milk of sheep is massaged in the animal to treat dislocation and deformities of bones. Sheep milk is poured in the animal eye to treat conjunctivitis.

Tribals of Rajasthan use animals and products derived from animals for treating various veterinary diseases. About 29 animal species, including 21 wild animals and birds are used for treating various veterinary diseases. In majority of such cases, blood was most commonly used product for treating body pain, arthritis, and healing the fractured bone of animals. Some of the respondents also mentioned about the use of spider web and powder of *Sambar* antler to treat the eye ailments of livestock. Whenever, needed, villagers purchase the antler of *Sambar* from local market. The boiled flesh of some of the marine fishes is also used by the locals to treat the foot and mouth disease of livestock, which is a very common disease in the area, while powder of *Ghoda Machchh*, probably sea horse, is used to treat the stomachache of horses.

The animal based medicines have always played a significant role in the healing practices, magic rituals, and religions of indigenous and western societies all over the world (Angeletti *et al.,* 1992 and Rosner, 1992).

However, as compared to the ethnobotanical documentation, the therapeutic use of animals and animal products to treat common human and domestic animal ailments have been little researched. There have been sporadic attempts within the country on the documentation of animal based traditional medication system (Pandey, 1996 ; Dutta *et al.,* 1996; Ghose & Maiti, 1996 and MoEF, 1996).

Though the present study is perhaps the first ever attempt to document the traditional ethnozoological knowledge of local communities in Rajasthan, further attempts are required to have a better understanding on the subject. Moreover, it was felt necessary because during interviews at some places respondents were not very open about the use of some more wild animals, probably because of their awareness of such act being illegal under the forest conservation laws.

Another important aspect of this study, which needs to be mentioned, is that the findings regarding the use of animals for medicines are purely based on the traditional beliefs of local communities and none of these animal based medicinal prescriptions has been authenticated or tested during the course of the study. Nevertheless, the healing properties of some of the animal products have been proved scientifically in the past (Sharma, 1996; Rosner, 1992 and Tajuddin & Amin, 1990) yet this aspect of traditional health care system needs further research not only to confirm the medicinal value of such animal based remedies, but also to facilitate more ecologically and socially sound development (Neto, 1999).

From ecological point of view, present study holds importance because some of the animals used by the locals for medicinal and other purposes are vulnerable or endangered or facing severe threats due to several kinds of anthropogenic pressures operating in the region (Geer and Guide, 2001). It is important to mention here that species such as Indian Wild Ass and Common Indian Monitor Lizard are listed as endangered while *Chinkara*, Indian Flap Shell Turtle and Peafowl are listed as vulnerable in the Red Data Book of Indian Animals (Red Data Book, 1994). Situation like this emphasizes the need of conservation programme for such species to be properly formulated and implemented. The existence of these animals is not only threatened by hunting for various purposes mentioned above but also because of the loss of habitats and other anthropogenic pressures. It is more important in view of the fact that if the remedial measures, for which these animals are used, are not proved scientifically, the common man should be made aware of this, which in future will significantly help in conservation of rare and endangered animals. The local people who hold the traditional ethnozoological knowledge can be roped in for implementation of participatory conservation programmes for such animals.

CHAPTER 6

ETHNOVETERINARY REMEDIES: MINERALS

During the ethnoveterinary survey, the authors also noted that besides the plants, animals and products of animal origin, the tribals also use minerals to treat the diseases of their animals. Most of these minerals are easily available at home. Following are such minerals arranged alphabetically followed by their local name in italics:

Alum / Alumen *Fitkari*

Characters: Colourless, transparent, crystals with acid, sweetish astringent taste.

Mode of administration: It is astringent, caustic, haemostatic, antispasmodic and antiseptic. Alum of potassium is given to animal to treat leucorrhoea, haematuria, haemoptysis, menorrhagia, gastric and intestinal catarrh/diarrhoea and other haemorrhages. It is applied externally on the skin of animal to treat skin inflammation. 1 kg. gum of *Cyamopsis tetragonoloba,* 1 kg. alum ($KAl(SO_4)_2.12.H_2O$) and 0.5 kg. common salt are mixed and heated with cow urine and about 100 ml of this solution is given to animal empty stomach to treat placental disorder. A mixture of seed oil of *Brassica campestris,* 5 g rhizome of *Curcuma longa* and 2 g potash alum is given to the animal orally through a drenching tube to treat internal wound. About 100 g of dried rhizome powder of *Curcuma amada* is mixed with 100 g of rock salt (NaCl), 100 g of alum, 100 g of *Piper longum,* 100 g seeds of *Trachyspermum ammi,* 250 g jaggery and 100 g milk fat. This mixture is divided in 3 parts. One part is given once in a day for 3 days to treat gynaecological problems after delivery, especially disposal of placenta after delivery.

Ammonium chloride (Ammoni chloridum) *Navasara, Chulika lavana, Navasadara*

Characters: White granular powder or lumps

Mode of administration: It is diuretic, relieves hepatic congestion and expectorant. Ammonium chloride is given to animal to treat hepatitis, pneumonia, fever and liver diseases. Sodium chloride is added in the seed oil of *Sesamum indicum* and used for massage to treat eczema. About 2 litre sesamum-oil, ½ kg roots of *Ziziphus mauritiana*, 100 g Ammonium chloride, 2 kg sugar and 100g clay is mixed with wheat husk and water is added and kept in an earthen pot upto three days and 750 ml of this mixture is given orally to the animal once in a day to induce lactation.

Calcium carbonate (Calcii carbonas) *Chalk, Vilati chuna*

Characters: Chalk occurs in irregular, white, amorphous pieces, sometimes as a powder.

Mode of administration: It is antacid- absorbent, desiccant and internally neutralizes the free acid of the gastric juice. Calcium carbonate is used to treat dyspepsia and checks sour eructation in animals. To treat burns in the animal the application of a mixture of chalk and linseed or olive oil is used. To treat discharges from ulcers, in combination with burnt coconut shell is useful. Internally it is used to treat irritant diahrroea. It coats and soothes the intestinal mucous membrane.

Calcium hydroxide (Lime) *Slaked lime churna, Churna*

Characters: Calcium hydroxide occurs in irregular, white, amorphous pieces/powder.

Mode of administration: It is astringent and antacid. Paste of lime is applied externally to treat tumours and warts in animal. Lime water is used to treat inflammatory swellings, in pruritis and distressing irritation of the genital organs, leucorrhoea and other vaginal discharges, syphilitic ulcers. Lime water given internally forms a good antacid. Used in pruritus irritation of the genital organs. To treat burns and scalds lime liniment called Carron oil, composed of equal part of lime water and a bland oil or olive oil or sesamum oil is applied.

Calcium sulphate (Calcii Sulphas) *Plaster of Paris, Sufed Phathar*

Characters: Dirty white amorphous powder.

Mode of administration: Plaster of paris is cooling, antacid and astringent. Useful to treat menorrhagia, inflammation around the ear and ottorhoea in animals. Plaster of paris is used as plaster to treat bone fracture.

Charcoal (Carbo ligni) *Lakrika-koyala*

Characters: Black moderately soft lumps. Powder charcoal is black amorphous powder.

Mode of administration: Deodorized, corrects bad odour, dry charcoal has the power of condensing oxygen with in its pores which then becomes a powerful deodorant, rapidly destroying organic substances. Charcoal is used to treat foul smelling diarrhoea in animals.

Copper sulphate *Nilatutia*

Characters: Occurs as blue crystalline masses.

Mode of administration: Powder of copper sulphate is used to treat epistaxis, chronic diarrhoea, dysentery and in various forms of bleeding from mucus membrane. Its mild lotion is used as nasal douche in respiratory diseases.

Ferrous sulphate (Iron rust) *Hara tutia*

Characters: Pale bluish green rhombic prism like crystals.

Mode of administration: It is haemostatic, tonic and astringent. Mild lotion of ferrous sulphate is used to treat epistaxis, and in various forms of bleeding from mucus membrane in animals.

Hydrochloric acid (HCl) *Tejaab, Namak ka tejaab*

Characters: Yellow liquid.

Mode of administration: Mixture of 50 ml hydrochloric acid (HCl), 50 ml latex of *Calotropis procera* and 50 ml latex of *Mangifera indica* is prepared and used as an antidote to scorpion bite.

Kaolin, Kaolinum *Gairika*

Characters: Occurs in irregular, white, amorphous pieces/ powder.

Mode of administration: Kaolin is used to treat chronic diarrhoea, dysentery, epistaxis, and in various forms of bleeding from intestinal mucous membrane.

Potassium nitrate *Yavakshar*

Characters: Occurs in irregular, white, amorphous pieces/ powder.

Mode of administration: Potassium nitrate is given to animal to treat dysurea, dropsy, acute rheumatism, bleeding from lungs and other internal organs and fever.

Silicate of magnesia *Shankh jiram*

Characters: Occurs in irregular, white, amorphous pieces/ thick masses. It forms a smooth powder, unctuous to touch, yielding a smooth slippery powder.

Mode of administration: It is powerful astringent, desiccant and styptic. Silicate of magnesia is used to treat diarrhoea, dysentery, menorrhagia, and leucorrhoea in animals. Its ointment is applied externally to treat wounds while paste on burns and scalds of the animals.

Sodium borate (Borax) *Sohaga*

Characters: It is composed of boric acid and soda. It exists as crystalline tough masses or in the form of translucent irregular masses. The colour is greyish-white, on exposure it becomes opaque or dirty white. It has a faintly balsamic odour and tastes like 'papada khar'.

Mode of administration: It is antacid. Borax is given to the animal to treat all sorts of phlegmatic complaints from common catarrh to bronchitis and pneumonia even attended with discharges from the ears and the nose. Externally borax is used to treat allay itching in urticaria, psoriasis, purulent wound and ulcers in animals. To treat sore nipples and other skin eruptions in animals, a solution of borax (1:8) is applied. It may also be employed in form of ointment in (1:8) ghee.

Sodium bicarbonate *Khane ka Soda, Khavano Soda*

Characters: White amorphous powder.

Mode of administration: Sodium bicarbonate is used to treat dyspepsia, tympani, diarrhoea, flatulence and urinary diseases. Used to treat rheumatism and ephemeral fever. Externally applied with water to relieve urticarial irruption and honey bee stings. About 50 g fruits of *Terminalia chebula*, 50 g rock salt, 50 g seeds of

Trachyspermum ammi, 25 g seeds of *Cuminum cyminum*, 25 g *Elytaria cardamomum* (chhoti ilaychi), 50 g sodium bicarbonate and 500 g jaggery is mixed and bolus of 150g of this mixture is given orally for three days to treat gastro intestinal disorders.

Sodium chloride (Common salt) *Lavan, Namak, Lun*

Characters: Transparent cubes or colourless crystalline grains and saline taste. Depending on the origin, salt is classified into the following types:

Ocean salt: Contains some iodine

Rock salt : Sindhaloon

This type of salt is obtained from earth mines as lumps of rocks or granular masses and is used as common salt. The big lumps are kept as animal licks on the manger.

Black salt: Kala loon

This type of salt is obtained from earth mines as lumps of rocks especially from Punjab and is used as saline sulphur and carminative and as condiment. It is also mixed in animal licks.

Mode of administration: It is antiseptic, deodorant, controls blood fluidity and body water. Isotonic, hyper and hypotonic solutions are used in different treatments. Mixed with magnesium chloride as saline purgative. Externally its saturated solution is used to treat boils.

Sulphur *Gandha and amlasar gandhaka*

Characters: Occurs in semi-transparent crystals.

Mode of administration: Bitter astringent taste with a peculiar strong smell. Acts as a laxative and alterative, diuretic and insecticide small doses, absorbed and may be detected in the sweat, stimulant to the membranes, specific action on the rectum and increases the haemorrhodial secretions. Sulphur is used to treat diseases like haemorrhoids, in chronic skin diseases etc. it is used both internally and externally. Internally it is given with milk. Applied externally in skin diseases, in 1:8 ointment. Sulphur is mixed with oil of *Brassica campestris* and applied on the body of animal to all kinds of skin diseases.

Zinc oxide *Putty*

Characters: White sticky amorphous powder.

Mode of administration: It is astringent and antiseptic, soothing, desiccant. As a powder dusted over eczema, impetigo, excoriations, bed sores and cracked nipples; as ointment applied to wounds, burns, vesicular eczema, chronic skin diseases internally act as nervine tonic, sedative, antispasmodic and astringent.

Plants constitute the mainstay of the folk-veterinary regimen but there are few mineral derived preparations which are also used by the tribals to treat various veterinary diseases. The present study report 17 minerals which are used by the tribals to prepare several remedies to cure veterinary diseases, hitherto not reported.

Besides plants, animals and mineral based remedies tribals of Rajasthan also use other stream of remedies such as cauterization, spirit medium etc. to cure the animals. Cauterisation (destruction of tissue by heat) is used in many cultures and countries such as the Fulani in Kenya and the Oromo stock raisers in Ethiopia. The Lozi in Zambia treat eye infections by cauterising the area around the eye (Beerling *et al*, 1988). Cauterisation on the chest for treatment of lung problems was observed by Anzuino (1999) in sheep in Somaliland.

Cauterisation is a practice with a long historical tradition common to traditional healers the world over. "Often frowned upon by conventional veterinary surgeons for its apparent cruelty and futility, the swear by this method [for treatment of disease in their animals and in themselves]" (Köhler-Rollefson, 1997). It is a highly complex system with possible parallels with acupuncture (Köhler- Rollefson, 1997).

Like *Ghuni*, firing healers frequently belong to pastoral communities and own animals themselves, they also treat both human beings and animals. More then half of all the respondents said to go to a firing healer in case of sickness. It is mostly applied to animals that have sprains or bruises but abscesses, nervous problems, coughing, liver flukes, udder problems and uncoordinated movement were also mentioned as reasons to go to a firing healer. Firing healers did not learn the profession from his father but from other people. They do not charge money because it is a god given profession. Location of the cauterisation point is associated with the location of the disease or problem. Animals suffering from ear infection are cauterised just behind the ear, rheumatism is treated by firing on the affected joints, eye problems are treated by cauterisation around the eyes. Timpani is treated by cauterisation of the flank of an animal and lung problems are treated by firing on the chest and cauterisation of one point on the head, the last is used when animals are coughing up blood. To enhance oestrus in an animal a point just below the anus is cauterised. Cauterisation "patterns" are not only point's but stripes, crosses and triangular forms are also used. Instruments for cauterisation are mostly old cooking utensils or pieces of metal.

During ethnoveterinary survey of the tribal area of Rajasthan it was found that livestock keepers will much rather resort to their own resources and experience, consult a traditional healer or, if all else fails, they visit a spirit medium.

The *Bhopa* is a spirit-medium, i.e. a person in whom a god becomes manifest after he has aroused himself in a state of trance. In this condition the *Bhopa* is endowed with supernatural powers and can provide help and give advice in important matters. Frequently, the *Bhopas* also belong to the pastoral castes. They may herd animals in daily life, but hold regular trance sessions at fixed days in the lunar cycle (LPPS, 1999). The *Bhopa* is visited mostly in the case of chicken pox, foot and mouth disease (FMD), but haematuria, liver fluke and sudden unexplained diseases are also reasons to visit the *Bhopa.* Some respondents visit the *Bhopa* for every sheep disease and consider it as part of a whole treatment complementing it with home made remedies.

The majority of respondents said that there is only one treatment for *Mata*. Because *Mata* is perceived as being caused by *Mataji;* a *Bhopa* (spirit medium) is visited and sometimes *mantras* and *Tantras* are being chanted. Ninety percent of all respondents applied a traditional vaccine in order to prevent the disease. Additionally, contact between healthy and sick sheep is avoided (60%), healthy sheep are taken out of the infected area for 30 days (3%) and women in their menstruation period are not allowed near sick sheep to prevent the disease from getting worse (51%). The function of the last is not really clear but the same rule is applied for Hindu temples in India, women in their menstruation period are not allowed inside. Since *Mata* is caused by a Hindu goddess there must be some sort of parallel between the two phenomenon's. When somebody heard that in a neighboring village sheep are infected with sheep pox the sheep in the village will be vaccinated as soon as possible.

There is no treatment for FMD but animals can be helped to recover. Plenty of water, shade and extra food help the animal to recover quickly. Local antiseptic treatments of the lesions together with antibiotic treatment help to stop the blisters getting infected by bacteria. Although only 20% claimed that *Khurpak* is caused by something supernatural no less than 67% of respondents applied magico-religious rituals to treat *Khurpak*, these included burning items of animal origin in the middle of the animal herd making sure that the smoke is spread over all the sheep. Items included donkey hoof, dog's and jackal's feces, lizards, turtle heads and birds. Furthermore mantras and *Tantras* are being chanted, a spirit medium is being visited and holy water collected from a temple is spread over the sheep while chanting mantras. It was very difficult to understand the meaning of these rituals and in many cases respondents replied that they were past down from their fathers but the meaning of the rituals was unclear to some of them. One explanation was that because the Brahmins (who to the perception of most respondents cause *Khurpak*) are vegetarians the burning of animal items would "scare" them off and the disease would leave the animals. A Similar situation described in literature concerns cattle; as an FMD prophylaxis, people may drench the cattle with wine in the belief that the wine will keep the disease away, just as good Brahmins avoid alcohol (Honey Bee, 1991). More then half of all respondents treat the wounds and lesions by applying oil and turmeric, Potassium permanganate dissolved in water, oil with salt, boiled ghee and a mixture of ghee, oil, salt and charcoal.. Additionally 50% of the respondents drench the sheep with oil and turmeric or ghee and turmeric in order to help the animal recover more quickly.

REFERENCES

Alawa, J.P., Jokthan, G.F. and Akul, K. (2002). Ethnoveterinary medical practice for ruminants in the subhumid zone of Northern Nigeria. *Preventive Veterinary Research*, 54: 79-90.

Ali, S.A.M. and Mahdihassan S, Bazar (1961). Medicines of Karachi: The drugs of animal origin. *Medicus,* 23: 72.

Almeida, M.R. (1998-2004). Flora of Maharashtra. Vol. (1-IV). *Blatter Herbarium, St. Xavier's College,* Mumbai.

Angeletti, L. R., Agrimi, U., Curia, C., French, D. and Mariani-Costantini R. (1992). Healing rituals and sacred serpents. *The Lancet*, 340: 223.

Anjaria, J., Parabia, M. and Dwivedi, S. (2002). Ethnovet Heritage Indian Ethnoveterinary - An Overview. *Pathik Enterprises*, Ahmedabad.

Anzuino, J. (1999). Investigation and Validation of Ethnoveterinary Medicine in the Context of the Community Animal Health Programme in Somaliland. An investigation sponsored by VETAID and submitted as a dissertation in partial fulfillment of the requirements of the Master of Science Degree in Tropical Veterinary Medicine. On-line document: http://vetaid.org/publications/mscomal/index.html

Anonymous (2004). Identification and evaluation of medicinal plants for control of parasitic of livestock. *Technical report. CIRG,* Makhdoom (Madhura).

Bachmann, F. (1998). Animal Recording for Livestock Development Experiences of the Swiss Agency for Development and Co-operation and of Interco-operation in India. *International workshop on animal recording for smallholders in developing countries,* Anand, India.

Beerling, M. (1988). Ten Thousand Kraals: Cattle and Ownership in Western Province, Animal Disease control Project Western Province, Mongu, Zambia, 60.

Bhandari M.M. (1990). Flora of Indian Desert, *Scientific Publishers (India)*, Jodhpur.

Blanca, E.I., Marica, M.J. and Morales, R. (1999). Medicinal veterinary plants of EI Caurel (Galicia, northwest Spain). *Journal of Ethnopharmacology,* 65: 113-124.

Coe, F.G. and Anderson, G.J. (1996). Ethnobotany of the Garifuna of Eastern Nicarague. *Economic Botany,* 50: 327-336.

Dwivedi, S.K. (1998). Overview of ethno-veterinary practices in India. ICAR Summer Short Course on techniques for scientific validation and evaluation of ethno-veterinary practices. Aug. 3-12, 1998, Division of Medicine, IVRI, Izatnagar, India: 1-5.

Dutta, A., Borkotoki, A., Kalita, J., Sharma, D.K. & Borthakur, S. (1996). Use of animals and animal produts in indigenous system of treatment in Assam, India, In: *Ethnobiology in Human Welfare*, edited by Jain S K, *Deep Publications*, New Delhi, 209.

Galav, P.K., Nag, A. and Katewa, S.S. (2007). Traditional herbal veterinary medicines from Mount Abu, Rajasthan. *Ethnobotany*, 19:120-123.

GEER and GUIDE, (2001). Ecological status of Narayan Sarovar Wildlife Sanctuary with a management perspective. Gujarat Ecological Education and Research (GEER) Foundation, Gandhinagar and Gujarat Institute of Desert Ecology (GUIDE), Bhuj.

Ghose, A.K. and Maiti P.K. (1996). Investigation of the animal drugs (mammals) used by the tribal people in India, in: Ethnobiology in Human Welfare, edited by Jain S K, *Deep Publications*, New Delhi, 200.

Honey Bee, (1991). Animal husbandry practices. In: *Honey Bee*: 2(1): 20-22.

Hooft, K., Van't (1995). Interface between local knowledge and western scientific knowledge in family level & extensive livestock keeping, *Utrecht*, Holland.

Hooker, J.D. (1872 – 1897). Flora of British India Vol. 1-7, *L. Reeve & Co., NR Ash food*, Kent.

International Network Prelude (2002). Available at: http:/www. Fundp.ac.be/prelude/index.htmo (last visited 27.06.2002).

Jain, Anita, Katewa, S.S., Choudhary, B.L. and Galav P.K. (2008). Traditional Herbal Veterinary Medicines from Tribal Area of Rajasthan, India. *Journal of Economic and Taxonomic Botany,* 32:264-269.

Jain, S.K. (1991). Dictionary of Indian Folk Medicine and Ethnobotany. *Deep Publications*, New Delhi.

Jain, S.K. (1999). Dictionary of Ethnoveterinary Plants of India. *Deep Publications*, New Delhi.

Joshi, P. (1995). Ethnobotany of primitive tribes in Rajasthan. *Printwell*, Jaipur, India.

Kadel, C. and Jain A.K. (2006). Plants used in ethnoveterninary practices in Jhabua district, Madhya Pradesh. *Ethnobotany,* 18(1&2):149-152.

Katewa, S.S. and Chaudhary, B.L. (2000). Ethnoveterinary survey of plants of Rajsamand district, Rajasthan. *Vasundhara,* 5: 95.

Katewa, S.S. and Jain, A. (2006). Traditional folk herbal medicines. *Apex Publishing House*, Jaipur.

Köhler-Rollefson, I. and Brauning, I. (1998). Anthropology veterinary medicine: The need for indigenizing the curriculum. The Ninth International conference of Institution of Tropical Veterinary medicines & animal Health production for Development, Harare, Zimbabwe.

Köhler-Rollefson, I. (1997). Between Burning Irons and Antibiotics: The significance of Ethnoveterinary Medicine. *German Research*, 2(3): 4-6.

Kumar, D. (2002). The use and relevance of Ethnoveterinary practices in sheep. *Indian Journal of Small Ruminants*, 8(2): 124-128.

Kumar, D. (2006). An approach for short-listing ethno-veterinary practices. *Livestock Research for Rural Development,* 18(5): Article 61.

Kumar, S., Goyal, S. and Parveen, F. (2004). Ethnoveterniary plants in Indian arid zone. *Ethnobotany,* 16(1&2): 91-95.

Khoda, V.K. (2005). Current priorities for the use of ethnoveterinary medicine in production of quality milk. *Proceedings of National conference on contemporary relevance of Ethnoveterinary medical traditions of India.* (Ed.) M.N.B. Nair, FRLHT, Banglore.

L.P.P.S. (1999). NGOs and Animal Health. A resource and tool kit for NGOs in Rajasthan/India. *Proceedings of a workshop held in Sadri* 13-15 March, 1999.

Lans, C., Harper, T., Georges, K. and Bridgewater, E. (2000). Medicinal plants used for dogs in Trinidad and Tobago. *Preventage Veterinary Medicine*, 45: 201-220.

Lans, C., Harper, T., George, K. and Bridgewater, E. (2001). Medicinal and Ethnoveterinary remedies of hunters and Trinidad. *BMC Complementary and Alternative Medicine*, 1: 10.

Livestock Census (2003). 17th Livestock Census. Department of Animal Husbandry, Dairying and Fisheries, Ministry of Agriculture, Government of India, New Delhi http://www.dahd.nic.in/

Mathias, E. (1996). How can ethnoveterinary medicine be used in field projects? In: *Indigenous Knowledge and Development Monitor*, 4(2): 6-7.

McCorkle, C.M. (1986). An introduction to ethnoveterinary research and development. *Journal of Ethnobiology*, 6(1):129-149.

McCorkle, C., Mathias, E. and Schilhorn van Veen T. (1996). Introduction: Ethnoveterinary Research & Development. In: Ethnoveterinary Research & Development, McCorkle, C., Mathias, E. and Schilhorn van Veen T. (Ed.), *Intermediate Technology Publications*. England.

Mini, V. and Sivadasan M. (2007). Plants used in ethnoveterinary medicine by Kurichya tribe of Wayanad district in Kerala, India. *Ethnobotany,* 19(1&2): 94-99.

MoEF (1996). All India Coordinated Research Project on Ethnobiology. Man and Biosphere Programme. *Ministry of Environment and Forests*, New Delhi.

Mokat, D.N. and Deokule, S.S. (2004). Plant used as veterinary medicine in the Ratanagiri district of Maharashtra. *Ethnobotany* 16(1&2): 131-135.

Nag, A., Galav, P.K., Katewa, S.S. and Swarnkar, S. (2009). Traditional herbal veterinary medicines from Kotda tehsil of Udaipur district (Rajasthan). *Ethnobotany*, (In press).

Nag, A., Galav, P.K. and Katewa, S.S. (2007). Indigenous Animal health care practices from Udaipur district of Rajasthan, India. *Indian Journal of Traditional Knowledge,* 6(4): 583-588.

Neto, E. M. C., (1999). Traditional use and sale of animals as medicines in Feira de Santana City, Bahia, Brazil. *Indigenous KnowledgeDevelopment Monitor*, 7:15.

Nfi, A. N., Mbanya, J. N., Ndi, C., Kameni, A., Vabi, M., Pingpoh, D., Yonkeu, S. and Moussa, C. (2001). Ethnoveterinary medicine in the Northern Province of Cameroon. *Veterinary Research Communications*, 25: 71-76.

Ole-Miaron, J.O. (2003). The Maasai ethnodiagnostic skill of livestock disease: a lead to traditional bioprospecting. *Journal of Ethnopharmacology*, 84: 79-83.

Pal, D.C. (1984). Observations on Ethnobotany of tribals of Subasiri, Arunachal Pradesh, *Bulletin of Botanical Survey of India,* 26: 26-37.

Pandey, V. N., (1996). The products of animal origin as recipes in Ayurvedic medicaments. in: Ethnobiology in Human Welfare, edited by Jain S.K., *Deep Publications*, New Delhi, 203.

Pieroni, A., Howard, P., Volpato, G., and Santoro, R.F. (2004). Natural remedies and Nutraceuticals used in Ethnoveterinary practices in Inland southern Italy, *Veterinary Research Communication,* 28(1): 55-80.

Puri, H.S. (1970). Drugs of animal origin used in Indian systems of medicine, *Nagarjun*, 13: 21.

Pushpangdan, P. (1990). Animal and animal products in the local health traditions in India, *Proceeding IInd International Congress on Ethnobiology*, 189.

Reddy, K.J. and Sudarshanam, G. (1987). Plants used as veterinary medicine in Chittoor district of Andhra Pradesh, India, *Int. J. Crude Drug Res.* 25 (3): 145-152.

Rosner, F. (1992). Pigeons as a remedy (*segulah*) for jaundice, *New York State J. Medicine*, 92: 189.

Scarpa, G.F. (2000). Plants employed in traditional veterinary medicine by the Criollos of the Northwestern Argentinc Chaco. *Darwiniana,* 38: 253-265.

Sebastian, M.K. and Bhandari, M.M. (1984). Some plants used as veterinary medicine by Bhils. *Int. J. trop. Agri,* 2: 307-310.

Sharma M.P. (1996). Drugs of animal origin in Unani medicine: The need for scientific evaluation, in: Ethnobiology in Human Welfare, edited by Jain S K, *Deep Publications*, New Delhi, 206.

Sharma, S. and Tiagi B. (1979). Flora of North-East Rajasthan. *Kalyani Publishers,* New Delhi.

Shukla, M.R. (1950). Unani Chikitsa Sagar (Hindi), *Motilal Banarasi Das*, Varanasi.

Sikarwar, R.L.S., Bajpai, A.K. and Painuli, R.M. (1994). Plants used as veterinary medicine by aboriginals of Madhya Pradesh, India. *Int. J. Pharmacog*, 32 (3): 251-255.

Singh, V. and Shetty, B.V. (1987–1993). Flora of Rajasthan, Vol I-III, *Botanical survey of India*, Kolkata.

Singh, V. and Pandey, R.P. (1998). Ethnobotany of Rajasthan. *Scientific Publishers*, Jodhpur.

Sharma, A.K. (2005). Common reproductive problems of the Gaushalas and their management. Compendium of Lectures of National Conference on Utility of Gaushalas for Improvement and Conservation of Indigenous Cattle, December 27-28, 2005, *National Bureau of Animal Genetic Resources, Karnal*, India.: 21-26.

Swarup, D. and Patra, R.C. (2005). Perspectives of Ethnoveterinary medicine in veterinary practice. *Proceedings of National conference on contemporary relevance of Ethnoveterinary medical traditions of India.* (Ed.) M.N.B. Nair, FRLHT, Banglore.

Tajuddin Y. and Amin K.M. (1990). The scientific evaluation of *Castoreum*: A drug of zoological source. *Proceeding IInd International Congress on Ethnobiology*, 186.

The Red Data Book of Indian Animals Part-I, (1994). Vertebrata (Mammalia, Aves, Reptilia & Amphibia). *Zoological Survey of India*, Calcutta.

Tiwari, L. and Pande, P.C. (2006). Ethnoveterinary plants of Uttarkashi district, Uttranchal, India. *Ethnobotany,* 18(1&2): 139-144.

Uncini Manganelli, R.E., Camangi, R. and Tomei, P.E. (2001). Curing animals with plants: traditional usage in Tuscany (Italy). *Journal of Ethnopharmacology,* 78: 171-191.

Unnikrishnan, P.M. and Shankar, D. (2005). Ethnoveterinary medicine in Ayurvedic perspective. *Proceedings of National conference on contemporary relevance of Ethnoveterinary medical traditions of India.* (Ed.) M.N.B. Nair, FRLHT, Banglore.

Vohora, S.B. and Khan S.Y. (1979). Animal origin drug used in Unani Medicine. *Vikas Publishing House* Pvt. Ltd., New Delhi.

Wahid, A. and Siddiqui, H.H. (1961). A Survey of Drugs, *Institute of History of Medcine and Medical Research*, New Delhi.

Waller, P.J., Berns, G., Thamsborg, S.M., Sukura, A., Richter, S.H., Ingebrigsen, K. and Hoglund, J. (2001). Plants as de-worming agents of livestock in the Nordic countries: historical perspective, popular beliefs and prospects for the future. *Acta Veterinaria Scandinavica,* 42: 31-44.

Yadav, D.K. (2007). Ethno-veterinary practices: A boon for improving indigenous cattle productivity in Gaushalas. Livestock Research for Rural Development, 19 (6).

Index to Minerals along with their English and local name

Index to Zoological name of animals along with their English and local name:

Index to local name of plants

Index to Botaical name